THE HIPPOCAMPUS - NEUROTRANSMISSION AND PLASTICITY IN THE NERVOUS SYSTEM

THE HIPPOCAMPUS - NEUROTRANSMISSION AND PLASTICITY IN THE NERVOUS SYSTEM

PHILIPPE TAUPIN

Nova Biomedical Books
New York

For permission to use material from this book please contact us:
Telephone 631-231-7269; Fax 631-231-8175
Web Site: http://www.novapublishers.com

LIBRARY OF CONGRESS CATALOGING-IN-PUBLICATION DATA

Taupin, Philippe.
The hippocampus : neurotransmission and plasticity in the nervous system / Philippe Taupin.
p. ; cm.
Includes bibliographical references and index.
ISBN-13: 978-1-60021-914-6 (hardcover)
ISBN-10: 1-60021-914-4 (hardcover)
1. Hippocampus (Brain)--Physiology. 2. Neural transmission. 3. Neuroplasticity. 4. GABA. [DNLM: 1. Hippocampus--physiology. 2. Neuronal Plasticity--physiology. 3. Synaptic Transmission--physiology. 4. gamma-Aminobutyric Acid--physiology. WL 314 T227h 2007] I. Title.
QP383.25.T38 2007
612.8'25--dc22 2007029504

Published by Nova Science Publishers, Inc. ✦ New York

CONTENTS

PREFACE

The hippocampus, greek name for seahorse, is one of the most fascinating and intriguing region of the mammalian brain. It is a bilateral incurved seahorse-shaped structure of the cerebral cortex. The hippocampus has a highly distinctive morphology. It is composed of two regions, the dentate gyrus (DG) and the Cornu Ammonis (CA). The nerve cells of the main layer of the DG and CA regions, the granule cells and pyramidal cells respectively, are organized in a tri-synaptic lamellaire circuit. The granule and pyramidal cells are glutamatergic excitatory. The granule cells elicit unique histological, biochemical, developmental, physio- and pathological features. The hippocampus is also an area of the brain that elicits a high degree of plasticity, like synaptic and phenotypic plasticity. It is also one of the few regions of the brain where neurogenesis, the generation of new nerve cells, occurs throughout adulthood. The hippocampus is involved in physio- and pathological processes, like learning and memory, Alzheimer's disease and epilepsy. For these reasons, the hippocampus is one of the most studied and characterized regions of the mammalian brain.

This book covers all the aspects of the hippocampus; its anatomy, histology, biochemistry, development, plasticity, physio- and pathology. It exposes the latest research and discoveries, particularly in adult neurogenesis and neural stem cell research. These discoveries considerably contribute to enhance our knowledge and understanding of the nervous system, and will shape future therapies for the treatment and cure of a broad array of neurological diseases, disorders and injuries, including Alzheimer' and Parkinson diseases, depression, cerebral strokes, spinal cord and traumatic brain injuries.

INTRODUCTION

The hippocampus (greek *hippocampus*: seahorse), is a bilateral incurved seahorse-shaped structure of the cerebral cortex [1]. The cerebral cortex also named "grey matter", as it is composed of neurons with unmyelinated fibers, is involved in a number of higher functions, like consciousness, information processing, language, memory and sensation.

The hippocampus is phylogenetically amongst the oldest structures of the brain. It lies beneath the neocortex, on the basal medial surface of the temporal lobes. The neocortex is the outer region of the cerebral cortex. It is composed of several lobes and has developed considerably during evolution in higher mammals. In rat and other lower mammals, it is a smooth structure, whereas in primates and other higher mammals, it has deep grooves and wrinkles. The neocortex is phylogenetically the most recent structure of the brain.

The hippocampus belongs to the limbic (latin *limbus*: border) system. An ensemble of brain regions, forming a *limbus* in the cerebral cortex, involved in emotion and memory, that also includes the amygdala, hypothalamus, olfactory cortex and other nearby areas.

The hippocampus has a highly distinctive morphology. It is composed of two regions, the dentate gyrus (DG) and the *Cornu Ammonis* (CA). The CA region is itself divided in 3 subfields, CA1, CA2 and CA3 [2]. Each of these regions is composed of a main cell layer, the principal cell layer. The nerve cells of the principal cell layer of the DG are the granule cells and the nerve cells of the principal cell layer of the CA regions are the pyramidal cells. The granule and pyramidal cells are excitatory glutamatergic.

The hippocampus is anatomically simpler than most other regions of the brain. The granule and pyramidal cells are organized in unique pathway, a tri-synaptic circuit. The tri-synaptic circuit is organized in lamella along the hippocampus. The hippocampus is also an area of the brain that elicits a high degree of plasticity, like synaptic and phenotypic plasticity.

The axons of the granule cells, the mossy fibers (MFs), establish synaptic contacts with the pyramidal cells of the CA3 region. The granule cells and MFs elicit unique histological, biochemical, developmental, and physio- and pathological features. Particularly, in 1992, Sandler and Smith reported the presence of γ-aminobutyric acid (GABA)-immunoreactivity in the MF ending nerves [3]. GABA is the main inhibitory neurotransmitter and the neurotransmitter of interneurons in the nervous system. The presence of an inhibitory neurotransmitter, in an excitatory nerve cell population, raises the question of the role of GABA in granule cells and MFs.

In the nervous system, a principle, known as the Dale's principle, enounces the principle of chemical identity of nerve cells [4]. The presence of GABA in granule cells raises the question of whether all MF synapses contain the same distribution of neurotransmitters and challenges basic concept of neuronal network functioning.

The hippocampus is also a site of a novel form of plasticity, the generation of new neuronal cells in the adult brain or adult neurogenesis [5]. The confirmation that neurogenesis occurs in the adult brain and neural stem cells reside in the adult central nervous system is as important for cellular therapy, as for our understanding of brain functioning and physiopathology [6].

The hippocampus is involved in physio- and pathological processes, like learning and memory, Alzheimer's disease and epilepsy.

In all, the hippocampus is one of the most fascinating and intriguing regions of the mammalian brain. Research and discoveries conducted in this brain region contribute considerably to enhance our knowledge and understanding of the nervous system. They will shape future therapies for the treatment and cure of a vast array of neurological diseases, disorders and injuries, including Alzheimer' and Parkinson diseases, depression, cerebral strokes, spinal cord and traumatic brain injuries.

REFERENCES

[1] Ramon y Cajal S. *Histologie du Système Nerveux de l'Homme et des Vertébrés*, Vols. 1 and 2. A. Maloine. Paris (1911).

[2] Lorente de No R. (1934) Studies on the structure of the cerebral cortex. II. Continuation of the study of the ammonic system. *J Psychol Neurol (Lpz). 46*, 113-77.

[3] Sandler R, Smith AD. (1991) Coexistence of GABA and glutamate in mossy fiber terminals of the primate hippocampus: an ultrastructural study. *J Comp Neurol. 303*, 177-92.

[4] Eccles JC. (1986) Chemical transmission and Dale's principle. *Prog Brain Res. 68*, 3-13.

[5] Altman J. (1962) Are new neurons formed in the brains of adult mammals? Science.135, 1127-8.

[6] Taupin P, Gage FH. (2002) Adult neurogenesis and neural stem cells of the central nervous system in mammals. *J Neurosci Res. 69*, 745-9.

Chapter I

THE HIPPOCAMPUS

ABSTRACT

The hippocampus (Greek. hippos, horse, and kampe, curve) is a highly distinctive and structured region of the brain. It is a compact, elongated and incurved structure, with a seahorse shape after which it is named. There are two hippocampi, located on each side of the brain. They lie beneath the neocortex, on the basal medial surface of the temporal lobes. The hippocampi are anatomically simpler than most other areas of the central nervous system (CNS). They are composed of two regions: the dentate gyrus (DG) and *Cornu Ammonis* (CA). The CA region is divided into four subfields, CA1, CA2, CA3 and CA4. The DG and CA contain a principal cell layer, the granule and pyramidal cell layers respectively. The hippocampi have a unique pattern of connectivity; a tri-synaptic circuit organized in lamella along their septotemporal axis. The entorhinal cortex represents the main afference of the hippocampus. The entorhinal cortex and hippocampus are an important memory center of the brain.

INTRODUCTION

The cerebral cortex is a highly developed structure of the human brain that plays a role in higher brain functions, like consciousness, information processing, language, memory and sensation [1]. It is part of the grey matter, composed of unmyelinated nerve cells. The neocortex is the outer region of the cerebral cortex. It is folded in lobes or cortical structures; the frontal, parietal, occipital and temporal lobes [2]. The hippocampus is a bilateral structure, located beneath the neocortex, on the basal medial surface of the temporal lobes (figure 1). It extends from the amygdala to the septum, along the temporal lobes [2-6]. The axis from the amygdala to the septum, along the temporal lobe, defines the septotemporal axis of the hippocampus. The hippocampus and subiculum, in the inferior part of the hippocampus, are often referred to as the hippocampal formation. The hippocampus is phylogenetically one of the most ancient structures of the brain. It receives its main afferences from the entorhinal cortex and sends efferences to other areas of the limbic and extra-limbic systems, like the fimbria/fornix and temporal neocortex. The hippocampus and entorhinal cortex represent an important memory center of the brain [1].

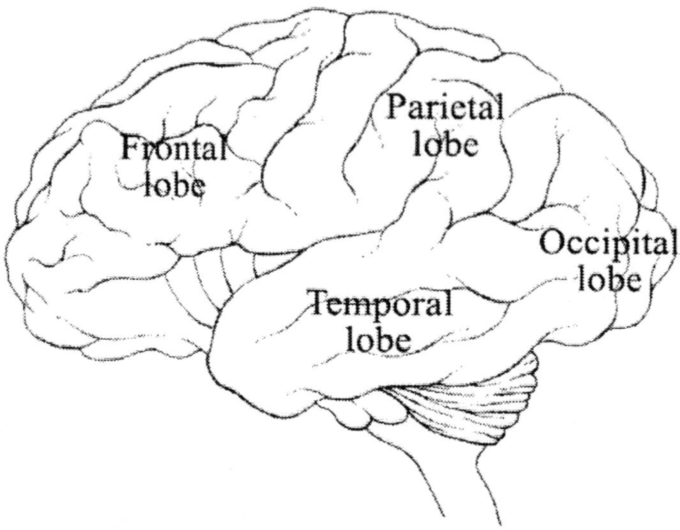

Figure 1. Schematic of the human cerebral cortex. The cerebral cortex is a highly developed structure of the human brain that plays a role in higher brain functions, like consciousness, information processing, language, memory and sensation. It is part of the grey matter, composed of unmyelinated nerve cells. The neocortex is the outer region of the cerebral cortex, it is folded in lobes or cortical structures; the frontal, parietal, occipital and temporal lobes. The hippocampus is a bilateral structure, located beneath the neocotex, on the basal medial surface of the temporal lobes. The hippocampus is phylogenetically is one of the most ancient structures of the brain.

THE HIPPOCAMPUS

The hippocampus is divided in two regions, the dentate gyrus (DG) and *Cornu Ammonis* (CA) or Ammon's horn [7]. The DG has a "V" or "U" shape. The CA is a curved structure forming a "U" enchased in the DG. The inside portion of the DG is known as the *hilus* or hilar region. Nissl and Golgi staining reveal that the DG and CA are each composed of a main cellular layer: the granule and pyramidal cell layers, respectively [8]. The granule and pyramidal cell layers extend all along the septotemporal axis of the hippocampus. Nissl stain is a histological stain that labels the rough reticulum endoplasmic of the cells (due to the staining of the ribosomal RNA). It stains all the cells, particularly the neurons and glial cells in brain sections. On nerve cells, Nissl stain is found in the cell bodies and dendrites, but absent from axons [9]. Cresyl violet is a Nissl stain that is widely used; it colors cell bodies in a brilliant violet. Golgi stain is a histological stain that labels only a few cell bodies in the tissue, but in their entirety. As such, it allows a detailed visualization of individual cells. This property makes this latter procedure particularly useful for characterizing neuronal cells and their extensions, neurites and axons [10].

The DG and CA are structured in layers or *strata*. From inside-out, the *strata* of the DG are: the polymorphic layer, the *stratum granulosum* and *stratum moleculare*. The polymorphic layer of the DG is located within the *hilus*. From inside-out, the *strata* of the CA are: the *stratum moleculare*, *stratum lacunosum* (or *lacunosum-moleculare*), *stratum radiatum*, *stratum lucidum*, *stratum pyramidale*, *stratum oriens* and the *alveus*. The principal layers of the DG and CA are the *stratum granulosum* and *pyramidale*, or granule and pyramidal cell layers, respectively. These dense layers contain the cell bodies of the granule and pyramidal cells. The polymorphic layer of the DG, the *stratum oriens* and *radiatum* of the CA regions contain various types of interneurons, mossy cells, basket cells, bipolar cells [11].

Hippocampal Subfields

The hippocampus is composed of anatomically distinct subfields, with different morphology, cell shape and size, connectivity, electrophysiological properties and susceptibility to insults [12-15].

The Dentate Gyrus

The granule cell layer or *stratum granulosum* is the principal layer of the DG; it contains the cell bodies of the granule cells. The somas of the granule cells have a diameter of approximately 7 μm. The *stratum moleculare* contains the proximal dendrites of the granule cells. The axons of the granule cells, the mossy fibers (MFs) project to the pyramidal cells of the CA region, known as the CA3 region [16]. The proximal sections of the MFs run through the polymorphic layer to the CA3 region. In the rat, the number of granule cells of the DG is estimated at approximately 1 million [17,18].

The Cornu Ammonis

The pyramidal cell layer or *stratum pyramidale* is the principal layer of the CA region; it contains the cell bodies of the pyramidal cells. Based on Golgi impregnation, Lorente de No (1934) divided the CA region into four subfields: CA1, CA2, CA3 and CA4 (figure 2). The CA1 region is adjacent to the subiculum. The CA3 region is adjacent to the fimbria/fornix and choroid plexus. The CA2 region is a small boundary between CA1 and CA3, and CA4 is located in the *hilus* of the DG [19]. Standard histological stains, like cresyl violet, delineate the cytoarchitectural boundaries of the hippocampal subfields, with the exception of the CA2/CA3 boundary. The hippocampal fissure is a cell-free natural division that separates the DG from the CA1 region.

The somas of the pyramidal cells have a triangular shape. Those in CA2 and CA3 are larger than those in CA1. They measure 40 to 60 μm at their base versus 20 to 40 μm for CA1 pyramidal cells. The *stratum oriens* contains the basal dendrites of the pyramidal cells. The *stratum moleculare* contains the apical dendrites of the pyramidal cells. The dendrites of CA3 pyramidal neurons are also thicker and shorter than those of CA1 pyramidal cells. The

MFs, the axons of the granule cells, project to the CA3 region and establish synaptic contacts with CA3 pyramidal cells in the *stratum lucidum*. The *stratum lucidum* is characterized by the so-called "thorny excrescences". The thorny excrescences correspond to the postsynaptic components of synapses between the MF terminals and the apical dendrites of CA3 pyramidal cells [16]. According to Lorente de No's (1934), the CA2 region corresponds to the region of the CA subfield that does not elicit the pattern of the *stratum lucidum* of CA3 with the so-called thorny excrescences and, thus, does not receive MF input [19]. The existence of CA2 has been questioned by other investigators. Many considered CA2 region as a small transitional zone between CA1 and CA3 without real identity, where the two classes of pyramidal neurons of CA1 and CA3 mingle [20-25]. According to these investigators, the CA region is primarily composed of two regions CA1 and CA3. Quantitative studies in rats estimate that the CA3 region is composed of 330.000 pyramidal cells and the region CA1 of 420,000 pyramidal cells. The number of interneurons is not known, but seems less important than the number of pyramidal cells [17,18].

HIPPOCAMPAL PATHWAYS

One of the main characteristics of the anatomy of the hippocampus is the connection of the main afference of the hippocampus with the cells of the principal layers, the granule and pyramidal cells, of the hippocampus in a lamellar tri-synaptic circuit. The hippocampus receives its afferences from various neighboring brain areas, like the entorhinal cortex, hypothalamus, septal nucleus median and nucleus of the diagonal band of Broca. Among them, the entorhinal cortex, an important area for memory in the brain, represents the main afference of the hippocampus.

The Tri-Synaptic Circuit

The hippocampus has a unique pattern of connectivity. The main pathways of the hippocampus are organized in a tri-synaptic circuit, in lamella along the septotemporal axis of the hippocampus (figure 2) [26-28]. The first link of the tri-synaptic circuit corresponds to the main afference of the hippocampus, the pyramidal cells of the layer II of the entorhinal cortex. Their axons, the perforant fibers, run through the *stratum moleculare* of the DG and project to the granule cells. Their axons are named perforant fibers, as they project to the granule cells through the hippocampal fissure, perforing it. The granule cells project their axons, the MFs, to the dendrites of the pyramidal cells of CA3, forming the second link of the circuit. The pyramidal cells of CA3 send collaterals, the collaterals of Schaeffer, to the pyramidal cells of CA1 forming the third link of the hippocampal tri-synaptic circuit. The collaterals of Schaeffer run through the *stratum radiatum*. The tri-synaptic organization of the main cell layers of the hippocampus implies that the information, from the entorhinal coxtex, flows through the hippocampus primarily unidirectionally. The tri-synaptic circuit is organized is near-transverse band or lamella, corresponding to a functional unit of the hippocampus. Lateral projections connect each lamella with each other along the septotemporal axis [26-28].

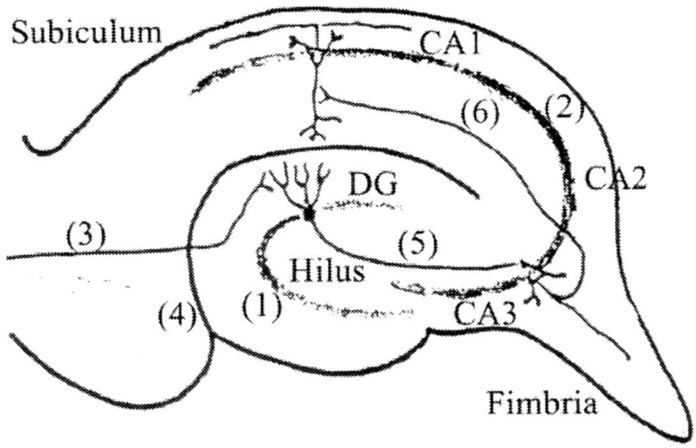

Figure 2. Schematic of a sagittal plan of the hippocampus. The hippocampus is a highly distinctive and structured region of the brain. It is a bilateral, compact, elongated and incurved structure. It is composed of two regions: the dentate gyrus (DG) and the *Cornu Ammonis* (CA). The DG has a "V" or "U" shape. The CA is a curved structure forming a "U" enchased in the DG. The *hilus* corresponds to the inside portion of the DG. The CA region is divided into four subfields: CA1, CA2, CA3 and CA4. The CA1 region is adjacent to the subiculum. The CA3 region is adjacent to the fimbria/fornix region. The CA2 region is a small boundary between CA1 and CA3. CA4 is located in the *hilus* of the DG. In the hippocampus, the identity of CA2 as a subfield of the CA region is the source of debates. The hippocampus has a unique pattern of connectivity. The cells of the principal layers of the DG and CA regions have distinctive morphologies, cell shapes, sizes and connections. The granule cell layer is the principal layer of the DG (1). The pyramidal cell layer is the principal layer of the CA (2). The main pathways of the hippocampus are organized in a tri-synaptic circuit, in lamella along the septotemporal axis of the hippocampus. The first link of the tri-synaptic circuit corresponds to the main afferences of the hippocampus, the pyramidal cells of the layer II of the entorhinal cortex. Their axons, the perforant fibers (3), project to the dentate granule cells through the hippocampal fissure. The hippocampal fissure is a cell-free natural division that separates the DG from the CA1 region (4). The granule cells project their axons, the mossy fibers (5), to the dendrites of the pyramidal cells of CA3, forming the second link of the circuit. The pyramidal cells of CA3 send collaterals, the collaterals of Schaeffer (6), to the pyramidal cells of CA1 forming the third link of the hippocampal tri-synaptic circuit. The tri-synaptic organization of the main cell layers of the hippocampus implies that the information, from the entorhinal cortex, flows through the hippocampus primarily unidirectionally. The tri-synaptic circuit is organized is near-transverse band or lamella corresponding to a functional unit of the hippocampus. Lateral projections connect each lamella with each other along the septotemporal axis. The fimbria/fornix is the main output of the hippocampus.

Besides the tri-synaptic network, where each region of the entorhinal cortex and hippocampus is linked to the next, a network of projections links one region to one or two regions upstream [29]. The axons of the pyramidal cells of the layer III of the entorhinal cortex, perforant fibers and temporo-ammonic projections, innerve the pyramidal neurons of the CA1 and CA3 regions. The CA3 pyramidal cells project not only to CA1, but also to the subiculum and entorhinal cortex, and sends axons, collateral fibers or recurrent fibers, to other neurons of CA3. The CA1 pyramidal cells also send fibers to the subiculum and entorhinal cortex. The only exception to this last rule concerns the granule cells of the DG that innervate only pyramidal cells of the CA3 region [30,31].

The axons of the pyramidal cells run through the *alveus* to the fimbria/fornix, the main output of the hippocampus.

Hippocampal Afferences

Besides the afferences from the entorhinal cortex, layers II and III, that project to the DG where they establish synaptic contacts with granule cells and to CA1 and CA3 pyramidal neurons, respectively, other afferences of the hippocampus originate from:

- the hypothalamus. These afferences project to the DG and CA2 regions [32,33]. These fibers enter the hippocampal formation by the fimbria/fornix,
- the septal nucleus median and nucleus of the diagonal band of Broca. These afferences project to all hippocampal regions, and mainly to the DG and CA3 regions [34,35]. These afferences, cholinergic and GABAergic, project to GABAergic interneurons, representing an example of double GABAergic inhibition in the septo-hippocampal network [36],
- the contralateral hippocampus. A network of afferent GABAergic fibers, the commissural fibers, originating from the contra-lateral hippocampus enters the other hemisphere via the *corpus callosum* and to the hippocampus via the fimbria/fornix. These fibers project mainly to the DG and run through the *stratum moleculare* of the DG [37,38]. There are other afferences of the hippocampus, like serotonergic, noradrenergic and possibly dopaminergic [29].

Hippocampal Interneurons

In the DG, the interneurons, mossy cells, basket cells, establish, via their axons, mostly symmetrical synaptic contacts with granule cells [39,40]. Symmetrical contacts are histological criteria indicative of inhibitory synapses. Afferences from the entorhinal cortex, the perforant path, that project to the DG where they establish synaptic contacts with granule cells, also establish synaptic contacts with interneurons in the DG molecular layer. These interneurons, in particular, send axonal projections throughout the subgranular zone, the layer beneath the DG [41,42].

In the CA regions, basket cells innervate the pyramidal cells with which they establish symmetrical synapses [43]. Lorente de No (1934) defined the CA4 region as located in the hilar region of the DG [19]. O'Keefe and Nadel (1978) reported that CA4 consists of CA3-like pyramidal neurons that do not receive inhibitory input from basket cells [12].

Feed-Back Inhibition and Feed-Forward Inhibition

In the CA regions, the basket cells that innervate the pyramidal cells with which they establish symmetrical synapses are innervated by commissural fibers and collateral fibers of pyramidal cells [44]. The commissural fibers and collateral fibers of pyramidal cells establish asymmetrical synapses with these interneurons [45]. Asymmetrical synapses are histological criteria indicative of excitatory synapses. The activation of the inhibitory interneurons is then controlled by pyramidal cells. The resulting inhibition is qualified recurrent "feed-back inhibition".

If the MFs innervate the pyramidal cells of CA3, most of these fibers and their collaterals innervate inhibitory interneurons [46,47]. The MFs establish synaptic contacts with inhibitory interneurons of the CA3 region and polymorphic layer of the hippocampus, characterized by the presence at regular interval (140 μm) of synapses, known as synapses "en passant" [46,47]. These MF endings establish asymmetrical synaptic contact at the level of the dendritic tree of interneurons (not at the level of the cell body) [46]. The activation of the inhibitory interneurons in CA3 region, by the MFs, induces an inhibition of the pyramidal cells. This control is qualified of "feed-forward inhibition" [48,49].

CONCLUSION

The hippocampus is composed of anatomically distinct subfields, with different morphology, cell shape and size, connectivity, electrophysiological properties and susceptibility to insults. Particularly, cytoarchitecturally discrete sub regions of the hippocampus can be distinguished from one another on the basis of morphology and neuronal network. In the hippocampus, the identity of CA2 as a subfield of the CA region is the source of debates.

The neuronal cells of the main cellular layers are primarily organized in a tri-synaptic mono-directional pathway. The tri-synaptic circuit has a lamellar organization, where the fibers are oriented parallel to each others and course nearly transversally to the long axis of the hippocampus, forming functional units of the hippocampus.

REFERENCES

[1] Kandel ER, Schwartz JH, Jessell TM. *Principles of Neural Science*. Publisher: McGraw-Hill Medical; 4 edition (January 5, 2000).

[2] Mai JK, Paxinos G, Assheuer JK. *Atlas of the human brain*. Publisher: Academic Press; 2 edition (December 2003).

[3] Paxinos G, Xu-Feng H, Toga AW. *The Rhesus monkey brain in stereotaxic coordinates*. Publisher: Academic Press (November 15, 1999).

[4] Wu J, Dubach MF, Robertson JE, Bowden DM, Martin RF. *Primate brain maps: structure of the Macaque brain*. Publisher: Elsevier (June 1, 2000).

[5] Paxinos G, Franklin KBJ. *The mouse brain in stereotaxic coordinates*. Publisher: Academic Press; 2 edition (November 2003).

[6] Paxinos G. *The rat brain in stereotaxic coordinates*. Publisher: Academic Press; 6 edition (December 18, 2006).

[7] Ramon y Cajal S. *Histologie du Système Nerveux de l'Homme et des Vertébrés*, Vols. 1 and 2. A. Maloine. Paris (1911).

[8] Amaral DG. (1978) A Golgi study of cell types in the hilar region of the hippocampus in the rat. *J Comp Neurol. 182*, 851-914.

[9] Nissl F. Ueber eine neue Untersuchungsmethode des Centralorgans zur Feststellung der Localisation der Nervenzellen. *Neurologisches Centralblatt, Leipzig. 13*, 507-8 (1894).

[10] Golgi C. *Sulla Fina Anatomia Deglia Orani Centrali del Sistema Nervoso*. Milano: U. Hoepli (1886).

[11] Altman J, Brunner RL, Bayer SA. (1973) The hippocampus and behavioral maturation. *Behav Biol. 8*, 557-96.

[12] O'Keefe J, Nadel L. *The hippocampus as a cognitive map*. Oxford: Oxford University Press (1978).

[13] Corsellis JA, Bruton CJ. (1983) Neuropatlology of status epilepticus in humans. *Adv Neurol. 34*, 129-39.

[14] Amaral DG, Insausti R. Hippocampal formation. In: *The human nervous system* (Paxinos G, ed), pp711-755. New York: Academic (1990).

[15] Storm-Mathisen J, Zimmerm J, Ottersen OP. *Progress in brain research*. Amsterdam: Elsevier Science Publishers B.V. (1990).

[16] Claiborne BJ, Amaral DG, Cowan WM. (1986) A light and electron microscopic analysis of the mossy fibers of the rat dentate gyrus. *J Comp Neurol. 246*, 435-58.

[17] Boss BD, Peterson GM, Cowan WM. (1985) On the number of neurons in the dentate gyrus of the rat. *Brain Res. 338*, 144-50.

[18] Amaral DG, Ishizuka N, Claiborne B. Neurons, numbers and the hippocampal network. *Progress in Brain Res. 83*, 1-11. J. Storm-Mathisen, J. Zimmer & O.P. Ottersen, eds. (1990).

[19] Lorente de No R. (1934) Studies on the structure of the cerebral cortex. II. Continuation of the study of the ammonic system. *J Psychol Neurol (Lpz). 46*, 113-77.

[20] Blackstad TW. (1956) Commissural connections of the hippocampal region in the rat, with special reference to their mode of termination. *J Comp Neurol.* 105, 417-537.

[21] Tole S, Christian C, Grove EA. (1977) Early specification and autonomous development of cortical fields in the mouse hippocampus. *Development. 124*, 4959-70.

[22] Swanson LW, Cowan WM. (1977) An autoradiographic study of the organization of the efferent connections of the hippocampal formation in the rat. *J Comp Neurol. 172*, 49-84.

[23] Zimmer J, Haug FM. (1978) Laminar differentiation of the hippocampus, fascia dentata and subiculum in developing rats, observed with the Timm sulphide silver method. *J Comp Neurol. 179*, 581-617.

[24] Gaarskjaer FB. (1986) The organization and development of the hippocampal mossy fiber system. *Brain Res. 396*, 335-57.

[25] Woodhams PL, Celio MR, Ulfig N, Witter MP. (1993) Morphological and functional correlates of borders in the entorhinal cortex and hippocampus. *Hippocampus. 3*, 303-11.

[26] Andersen P, Bliss TV, Lomo T, Olsen LI, Skrede KK. (1969) Lamellar organization of hippocampal excitatory pathways. *Acta Physiol Scand. 76*, 4A-5A.

[27] Amaral DG, Witter MP. (1989) The three-dimensional organization of the hippocampal formation: a review of anatomical data. *Neurosci. 31*, 571-91.

[28] Andersen P, Soleng AF, Raastad M. (2000) The hippocampal lamella hypothesis revisited. *Brain Res. 886*, 165-71.

[29] Brown T H, Zador AM. Hippocampus. In: *The synaptic organization of the brain*, Shepherd G.M. pp 346-388. ed. Oxford (1991).

[30] Blackstad TW, Kjaerheim A. (1961) Special axo-dendritic synapses in the hippocampal cortex: electron and light microscopic studies on the layer of the mossy fibers. *J Comp Neurol. 117*, 133-59.

[31] Hamlyn LH. (1962) The fine structure of the mossy fibre endings in the hippocampus of the rabbit. *J Anat. 96*, 112-20.

[32] Segal M. (1979) A potent inhibitory monosynaptic hypothalamo-hippocampal connection. *Brain Res. 162*, 137-41.

[33] Wyss JM, Swanson LW, Cowan WM. (1979) Evidence for an input to the molecular layer and the stratum granulosum of the dentate gyrus from the supramammillary region of the hypothalamus. *Anat Embryol (Berl). 156*, 165-76.

[34] Amaral DG, Kurz J. (1985) An analysis of the origins of the cholinergic and noncholinergic septal projections to the hippocampal formation of the rat. *J Comp Neurol. 240*, 37-59.

[35] Frotscher M, Leranth C. (1985) Cholinergic innervation of the rat hippocampus as revealed by choline acetyltransferase immunocytochemistry: a combined light and electron microscopic study. *J Comp Neurol. 239*, 237-46.

[36] Krnjevic K, Reiffenstein RJ, Ropert N. (1981) Disinhibitory action of acetylcholine in the rat's hippocampus: extracellular observations. *Neurosci. 6*, 2465-74.

[37] Frotscher M, Zimmer J. (1983) Commissural fibers terminate on non-pyramidal neurons in the guinea pig hippocampus -- a combined Golgi/EM degeneration study. *Brain Res. 265*, 289-93.

[38] Leranth C, Frotscher M. (1983) Commissural afferents to the rat hippocampus terminate on vasoactive intestinal polypeptide-like immunoreactive non-pyramidal neurons. An EM immunocytochemical degeneration study. *Brain Res. 276*, 357-61.

[39] Amaral DG. (1978) A golgi study of cell types in the hilar region of the hippocampus in the rat. *J Comp Neurol. 182*, 851-94.

[40] Seress L, Frotscher M. (1991) Basket cells in the monkey fascia dentata: a Golgi/electron microscopic study. *J Neurocytol. 20*, 915-28.

[41] Freund TF, Buzsaki G. (1996) Interneurons of the hippocampus. *Hippocampus. 6*, 347-470.

[42] Kneisler TB, Dingledine R. (1995) Spontaneous and synaptic input from granule cells and the perforant path to dentate basket cells in the rat hippocampus. *Hippocampus. 5*, 151-64.

[43] Mott DD, Turner DA, Okazaki MM, Lewis DV. (1997) Interneurons of the dentate-hilus border of the rat dentate gyrus: morphological and electrophysiological heterogeneity. *J Neurosci. 17*, 3990-4005.

[44] Frotscher M, Leranth C. (1988) Catecholaminergic innervation of pyramidal and GABAergic non-pyramidal neurons in the rat hippocampus: double label immunostaining with antibodies against tyrosine hydroxylase and glutamate decarboxylase. *Histochem. 88*, 313-9.

[45] Gamrani H, Onteniente B, Seguela P, Geffard M, Calas A. (1986) Gamma-aminobutyric acid-immunoreactivity in the rat hippocampus. A light and electron microscopic study with anti-GABA antibodies. *Brain Res. 364*, 30-8.

[46] Frotscher M. (1985) Mossy fibres form synapses with identified pyramidal basket cells in the CA3 region of the guinea-pig hippocampus: a combined Golgi-electron microscope study. *J Neurocytol. 14*, 245-59.

[47] Acsady L, Kamondi A, Sik A, Freund T, Buzsaki G. (1998) GABAergic cells are the major postsynaptic targets of mossy fibers in the rat hippocampus. *J Neurosci. 18*, 3386-403.

[48] Buzsaki G. (1984) Feed-forward inhibition in the hippocampal formation. *Prog Neurobiol. 22*, 131-53.

[49] Frotscher M. (1989) Mossy fiber synapses on glutamate decarboxylase-immunoreactive neurons: evidence for feed-forward inhibition in the CA3 region of the hippocampus. *Exp Brain Res. 75*, 441-5.

Chapter II

NEUROTRANSMITTERS IN THE NERVOUS SYSTEM

ABSTRACT

Chemical transmission is the main mode of transmission of nerve activity in the nervous system. It occurs at specialized structures, the synapses, and is mediated by neurotransmitters. Neurotransmitters are chemical substances or molecules that relay nerve activity between nerve cells or nerve cells and other cells, like muscle cells and glands. They are defined by a set of specific criteria that must be demonstrated for a substance to qualify as neurotransmitter. In the nervous system, different populations of nerve cells are believed to contain either an excitatory or inhibitory neurotransmitter, defining excitatory and inhibitory neurons, respectively. Glutamate (L-glutamic acid, Glu) is the main excitatory neurotransmitter and γ-aminobutyric acid (GABA) the main inhibitory neurotransmitter in the nervous system. Co-localization of Glu and GABA has been reported in various populations of nerve cells, underlying the existence of different pools of amino acids, neurotransmitter and metabolic.

INTRODUCTION

In the nervous system, nerve cells are connected to each other and non-neuronal cells through specialized structures which relay nerve activity, the synapses [1]. In 1921, Otto Loewi reported the first evidences that chemical substances underlie the transmission of nerve activity, leading to the identification of acetyl choline as the first neurotransmitter [2-3]. Since then chemical transmission has been shown to be the main mode of transmission of nerve activity, and various neurotransmitters and their mechanisms of action have been identified and characterized in the nervous system [4,5].

Neurotransmitters are chemical substances that relay the transmission of nerve activity. They are defined by a set of criteria. Neurotransmitters are synthesized and stored in nerve cells; they are stored in synaptic vesicles in the presynaptic terminals (or boutons) of the nerve endings. Neurotransmitters are released during nerve activity in the synaptic cleft; they are released in a calcium-dependent manner. They interact with specific receptors in the postsynaptic membrane to relay the transmission of nerve activity. Neurotransmitters are cleared from the synaptic cleft, once released, by uptake and/or degradation, inhibiting the activity of the neurotransmitter [6].

The transmission of nerve activity or synaptic transmission is mediated by the release of neurotransmitters from the presynaptic terminals and their interactions with postsynaptic receptors. According to the vesicular hypothesis of transmitter release, neurotransmitters are released from the presynaptic terminals by exocytosis of synaptic vesicles [7]. Other models of transmitter release have been proposed, like the plasmalemmal proteolipid mediatophore that also supports the quantal release of neurotransmitters at the synapse [8]. The uptake of neurotransmitters in the presynaptic terminals and synaptic vesicles is mediated by carriers in the plasma membrane and vesicular transporters, respectively. Uptake carriers in the plasma membrane and vesicular transporters have different properties; particularly, vesicular transporters are driven by an electrochemical proton gradient across the vesicle membrane [9].

Neurotransmitters belong to various classes of molecules, like amino acids, peptides and monoamines. Amino acids are the main neurotransmitters of the nervous system. Among them, there are four amino acids that act as neurotransmitters, Glu, aspartate (L-aspartic acid, Asp), GABA and glycine (Gly) [10,11].

Neurotransmitters in the Nervous System

Characterizing Neurotransmitters

A substance candidate neurotransmitter must fulfill the following criteria. It must be present in nerve cells from which it is released, it must be present in the nerve terminals and within synaptic vesicles. The nerve cells must express the biosynthesis enzymes for the substance, as well as the precursors and intermediaries of its biosynthetic pathway. The substance must be released from the nerve terminals during stimulation, in a calcium-dependent manner. The substance must act through receptors on the postsynaptic membrane. The mechanisms of inactivation, enzymes of degradation or membranous uptake carrier, of the transmitter must be characterized. When applied postsynaptically, the substance, its agonists or antagonists must mimic or inhibit the activity of the endogenous neurotransmitter [11].

Ionotropic and Metabotropic Receptors

There are two types of receptors of neurotransmitters, ionotropic and metabotropic. Ionotropic receptors are coupled to ion channels or ligand gated ion channels. The interaction of neurotransmitters with ionotropic receptors opens rapidly ion channels. The rapid opening of ion channels generates fast and large changes in the conductance of the membrane, leading to the depolarization or hyperpolarization of the membrane. Neurotransmitters acting on ionotropic receptors are qualified of fast-acting neurotransmitters. Metabotropic receptors are coupled to secondary messenger systems, like adenylate cyclase or protein G. The interaction of neurotransmitters with metabotropic receptors affects the metabolic state of the cells. Metabotropic receptors induce a slower response than ionotropic receptors, without significant changes in conductance and potential of the membrane [12].

The interaction of fast-acting neurotransmitters with ionotropic receptors is responsible for the transmission of the nerve activity, whereas the interaction of neurotransmitters with metabotropic receptors may mediate metabolic changes in the cells, as well as trophic activities. A neurotransmitter can act simultaneously on ionotropic and metabotropic receptors. Activities of neurotransmitters are therefore not limited to neurotransmission.

Excitatory and Inhibitory Neurotransmitters

In the nervous system, there are two types of fast-acting neurotransmitters, excitatory and inhibitory. Different populations of nerve cells are believed to contain either an excitatory or inhibitory fast-acting neurotransmitter, defining excitatory and inhibitory neurons, respectively [13]. Excitatory neurotransmitters depolarize the membrane potential of the target cells, decrease the conductance of the postsynaptic membrane and increase their excitability. This leads to the propagation the nerve activity. Inhibitory neurotransmitters hyperpolarize the membrane potential, increase the conductance of the postsynaptic membrane and decrease the excitability of the target cells. Inhibitory neurotransmitters inhibit the propagation of nerve activity by making nerve cells less responsive to excitatory inputs.

The organization of the network in excitatory and inhibitory neurons establishes the basis of the functioning of the nervous system: excitatory nerve cells produce short-latency excitation of postsynaptic target cells and inhibitory neurons control their excitability, and therefore nerve activity [13].

Glutamate and GABA the Main Neurotransmitters of the Nervous System

The first evidence that an amino acid, Glu, acts as a neurotransmitter in the nervous system was reported by Curtis et al. (1959). The authors showed that microiontophoretically-applied glutamate induces nerve activity on spinal neurons in brain slices [14]. The introduction and use of selective antibodies to study the immunohistochemical distribution of amino acids revealed that Glu is selectively enriched in excitatory neurons of the nervous system and their terminals [15]. The characterization and identification of the release of Glu from nerve terminals, of the localization of Glu within synaptic vesicles, of glutamate receptors (GluRs), of membranous and vesicular Glu transporters, and the introduction of pharmacological tools to study GluRs further contributed to characterize the role of Glu, as a neurotransmitter of the nervous system [16,17].

In mammals, Glu is the main excitatory neurotransmitter of the nervous system, as virtually all excitatory synapses are glutamatergic [18]. Other studies revealed that GABA is the main inhibitory neurotransmitters, particularly of interneurons [19,20].

In the hippocampus, the cells of the principal layers of the hippocampus, the granule and pyramidal cells, are excitatory glutamatergic, whereas the interneurons are inhibitory GABAergic [19-25]. The pyramidal cells of the layer II of the entorhinal cortex, the main afferences of the hippocampus, are also excitatory glutamatergic. Hence, the main pathway of the hippocampus, organized in a trisynaptic circuit, is glutamatergic and the information, from the entorhinal coxtex that flows primarily unidirectionally through the hippocampus, is excitatory [26-28].

THE EXCITATORY NEUROTRANSMITTER GLUTAMATE

Metabolism

The brain is enriched in Glu. This reflects its metabolic role, particularly in the glutamine (Gln) cycle. In the Gln cycle, Gln is synthesized from Glu in glial cells by the glial-specific enzyme, Gln synthetase. Gln diffuses from glial cells to nerve cells. In nerve cells, Glu is synthesized from Gln by glutaminase. Glu released during synaptic release is transported inside glial cells where it is metabolized in Gln [29]. Glu is also synthesized in nerve cells either by transamination of Asp by aspartate amino-transferase, and from 2-oxoglutarate by Glu dehydrogenase. Glucose, via the Krebs cycle, is the main source of 2-oxoglutarate. Glu is also an amino acid substrate for protein synthesis.

Glutamate Receptors

The introduction of agonists and antagonists of GluRs led to the identification and characterization of three classes of ionotropic GluRs and one class of metabotropic Glu-R [30]. Ionotropic GluRs are multimeric receptors composed of a combination of 4 to 5 subunits, GluR1 to 5. They are coupled to sodium and calcium channels. Ionotropic GluRs are classified in function of their main agonist. The N-methyl-D-aspartate (NMDA) receptor has for agonist NMDA. The α-amino-3-methyl-4-isoxazolepropionate (AMPA) receptor has for agonists, quisqualate and AMPA. The kainate receptor has for agonist kainic acid [31,32]. The NMDA receptor is blocked by a voltage-dependent blockage of the channel ion by magnesium. The activation of ionotropic GluRs mediates the opening of sodium and calcium ion channels. The influx of sodium and calcium inside the cells induces the depolarization of the membrane potential of the postsynaptic membrane, leading to the transmission of nerve activity [33]. The metabotropic receptors belong to the family of G-protein coupled receptors; they are activated by quisqualate and induce the formation of inositol triphosphate via a G-protein sensitive to pertussis toxin [33].

Glutamate Transporters

L-Glu, D- and L-Asp are transported inside nerve and glial cells, by high-affinity transporters in the plasma membrane that are coupled to the entry of sodium and potassium ions [34-36]. L-Glu is transported in synaptic vesicles by a low affinity vesicular transporter that is independent of the sodium gradient and depends of a proton pump coupled with an ATPase. The vesicular transporter for L-Glu does not transport Asp [37-39].

THE INHIBITORY NEUROTRANSMITTER GABA

Metabolism

GABA is a non-protein amino acids synthesized in the cytoplasm of neurons from Glu by Glu decarboxylase (GAD) and from Gln by glutaminase [40-42]. GAD catalyzes the decarboxylation of Glu to GABA and CO_2. GAD uses pyridoxal phosphate (PLP) as a cofactor [40,41]. The brain contains two forms of GAD, GAD65 and GAD67. They derived from two different genes [43,44]. They have different molecular weight, different interaction with PLP and different cellular distribution. GAD65 is mainly localized in the ending nerves, whereas GAD67 in mainly localized in the cell bodies and dendrites [43,45]. The GAD associated to PLP, named apo-GAD, is enzymatically inactive, while when GAD is associated to PLP, named holo-GAD, it is enzymatically active [46,47]. The interaction of GAD with PLP is the main factor of short-term regulation of GAD activity. In the brain, approximately 50% of GAD is apo-GAD and serves as a reservoir when additional GAD activity is required. The high proportion of inactive enzyme suggests its involvement in short-term adaptive response for GABA synthesis [48]. The expression of the two forms of GAD65 and 67 is regulated independently. GAD65 is mainly associated with synthesis of the neurotransmitter pool of GABA whereas GAD67 is mainly associated with synthesis of the metabolic pool of GABA [49].

GABA Receptors

An ionotropic receptor, the GABA-(A) receptor (GABA-(A)R), and a metabotropic receptor, the GABA-B receptor (GABA-(B)R), have been reported for GABA [50,51]. The GABA(A)-R is activated by isoguvacine and muscimol and is blocked competitively by bicuculline and picrotoxine [52]. The interaction between GABA and GABA-(A)R mediates the opening of chloride ion channels and the entrance of chloride ions inside the cells. The influx of chloride ions inside the cells induces hyperpolarization of the membrane potential of the postsynaptic membrane, leading to the inhibition of the transmission of nerve activity [53]. The GABA(B)-R are G-protein coupled receptors, activated by baclofen [54].

GABA Transporters

GABA and Gly are transported inside nerve and glial cells by a plasma membrane transporter coupled to the entry of ion sodium and potassium [55,56]. The presence of plasma membrane GABA transporter (GAT) is restricted to nerve cells that synthesize and release GABA and to glial cells [57-59]. Use of the blocker of GAT, tiagabine, during depolarization of neocortical neurons (GABAergic) with high concentration of potassium, like 55 mM K^+, in the presence of $Ca2^+$ allowed the study of GABA release selectively from the vesicular pool, prolonged K^+-evoked depolarization produces a reversal of the GABA plasma membrane transporters [55,56,60,61]. GABA and Gly are transported in synaptic vesicles by a vesicular transporter that depends on a proton pump coupled to an ATPase, the vesicular GABA transporter (VGAT) [62-64]. As such, VGAT is expressed in both GABAergic and glycinergic neurons.

Defining Glu and GABA as Neurotransmitters

GABA is thought to Occur in high Concentrations Exclusively in Nerve Cells that use it as Neurotransmitters

GABA, but also Gly are thought to be present in high concentrations exclusively in nerve cells that use them as neurotransmitters. GABA is produced by the 65- and 67-kDa forms of GAD [43,44]. The distribution of GAD65 and GAD67 underlies the regulation of metabolic versus neurotransmitter pools of GABA in those cells [48,49,65]. The detection of high concentration of GABA in nerve endings or the GABA synthesizing enzyme, GAD65, are therefore well accepted criteria to identify a population of nerve cells using GABA as neurotransmitter [44,66]. In support of this contention, GABA antibodies label selectively neuronal populations that are thought to be GABAergic [67]. In all, GABA is concentrated exclusively in neurons that use GABA as a transmitter. By inference, there are good reasons to assume that cells eliciting a strong GABA-immunoreactivity or GAD65-immunoreactivity are GABAergic neurons.

Glu is not Restricted to Neurons that use it as a Neurotransmitter

Glu is the main excitatory neurotransmitter of the nervous system [16-18]. In contrast to GABA, Glu is involved in protein synthesis. Glu is also involved in a series of metabolic reactions. Indeed, because Glu serves a variety of functions in the nervous system and is present in most or all cells compartment, it is one of most difficult substances to interpret as neurotransmitter [17]. Hence, Glu is not restricted to neurons that are thought to use it as a neurotransmitter, but occurs in varying amount in all cellular compartments in the brain. Particularly, numerous reports reveal that Glu-immunoreactivity is detected in various types of nerve cells assumed to use GABA, dopamine or serotonin as transmitters [67].

Numerous reports reveal the colocalization of Glu and GABA in cells known to use GABA as neurotransmitter. Colocalization of Glu and GABA immunoreactivities was reported in 25% of terminals of the locus coeruleus, a region involved in the sleep-wake cycle and regulation of attention and orientation behavior [68-70]. Colocalization of Glu and GABA was reported in some afferences of spinal motoneurones [71]. High levels of Glu-immunoreactivity were found within terminals of the rat rostral ventrolateral medulla that were strongly immunoreactive for GABA [70]. In the rat hindlimb motoneurons, 40% of GABA/Gly boutons contain Glu [72]. There are indeed numerous examples of colocalization of Glu- and GABA-imunoreactivities in nerve cells and their terminals in various other brain regions and species. For example, in the cortex [73], striatum [74], pulvinar-lateralis posterior complex [75], retina [75-79], cerebellum/cerebellar cortex [80,81], area postrema [82], in a population of neurons in the periglomerular region of the olfactory bulb [81], and in horizontal and amacrine cells in the retina of chicken, goldfish, lizard, tiger salamender and human [77,78,83-86]. Also, in neurons of the frog vestibular nuclear complex, the termination field of afferent fibers from the vestibular and auditory sense organs, [87], in a small population of neurons of the rat accessory olfactory bulb [88] and in a population of calbindin-immunoreactive terminals of the intermediolateral cell column of the spinal cord [89]. In all, there are numerous reports of the colocalization of Glu and GABA, particularly in GABAergic nerve cells and terminals.

Glu is a substrate for GABA synthesis; GABA is synthesized in the cytoplasm of neurons from Glu by GAD [40,41]. The detection of high concentration of GABA in nerve endings or the GABA synthesizing enzyme, GAD, are well accepted criterion to identify a population of nerve cells as using GABA as neurotransmitter. Colocalization of Glu and GABA in the same nerve cells or terminals does not necessarily imply that both amino acids are employed as neurotransmitters. Indeed, in GABAergic cells, the presence of Glu may reflect the use of Glu as a substrate for GABA synthesis. It may represent a metabolic rather than a transmitter pool of Glu [67,68,83-85]. The transmitter pool of Glu is assumed to be localized in synaptic vesicles. In GABAergic nerve cells, the colocalization of Glu and GABA may reflect, in most cases, the existence of a metabolic pool of Glu.

In some reports, like in the retina of tiger salamender and human, a population of amacrine cells elicits intense Glu-immunoreactivity compared to other species and similar in intensity to bipolar cells, in which Glu is likely transmitter [86]. In those cells, it is proposed that Glu may be in excess than that required for GABA synthesis and could be co-released with GABA. Glu may act as a neurotransmitter in amacrine cells of the retina of tiger salamender and human. This raises the possibility that Glu and GABA could co-released and both act as neurotransmitters in those cells [80,90-92]. The co-release of excitatory and inhibitory neurotransmitters would provide excitatory inputs to ganglion cells in addition to that provided by bipolar cells in the retina. Alternatively, the presence of high concentration of Glu in those cells could signify that they elicit a strong metabolism for GABA, requiring high level of Glu. Glu would serve a metabolic function [93]. The role of Glu in GABAergic nerve cells, eliciting unusually high levels of Glu-immunoreactivity, remains to be further clarified.

In all, Glu serves a variety of functions in the nervous system and is present in most or all cells compartment [17,18]. Nerve cells contain two pools of Glu: a metabolic and transmitter pool [45,84]. The existence of two pools of Glu interferes with the identification of Glu as a neurotransmitter in nerve cells. It is proposed that to qualify as transmitter, amino acids, and in particular Glu, should be found in high concentrations in areas of high vesicular density, i.e. within axon terminals. Whereas free amino acids with no transmitter role should be found more evenly distributed throughout the cytoplasm; they should not be specifically enriched in nerve terminals. This distinctive feature of transmitter versus metabolic pools of amino acids should be useful in distinguishing between amino acids transmitter and non-transmitter, particularly for Glu [81]. This shows that colocalization of Glu and GABA does not necessarily imply that both amino acids are employed as transmitters, particularly for Glu. Neurotransmitter pools of Glu must therefore be convincingly distinguished from metabolic pools of Glu. The detection of Glu in synaptic vesicles and physiological evidences of the involvement of Glu in synaptic transmission may define the transmitter identity of a cell population as using Glu as neurotransmitter, rather than a high concentration of transmitter substances or the presence of its biosynthetic enzymes [67].

Conclusion

Neurotransmitters are substances that relay nerve activity in the nervous system. The interaction of neurotransmitters with ionotropic receptors defines the nerve cells' phenotype. The organization of the network in excitatory and inhibitory neurons establishes the basis of the functioning of the nervous system. In the nervous system, Glu is the main excitatory neurotransmitters and GABA is the main inhibitory neurotransmitter. GABA is thought to be present in high concentrations exclusively in nerve cells that use them as neurotransmitters. By inference, there are good reasons to assume that cells eliciting a strong GABA-immunoreactivity or GAD65-immunoreactivity are GABAergic neurons. In contrast to GABA, Glu is present in most or all cells compartment, and is involved in protein synthesis and in a series of metabolic reactions. Glu is one of most difficult substances to interpret as neurotransmitter and physiological evidences of the involvement of Glu in synaptic transmission are required, to define the role of Glu, as a neurotransmitter. Numerous reports reveal the colocalization of Glu and GABA in nerve cells, particularly in GABAergic nerve cells. In those cells, the presence of Glu may reflect the existence of a metabolic pool rather than a neurotransmitter pool of Glu.

References

[1] Ramon y Cajal S. *Histologie du Système Nerveux de l'Homme et des Vertébrés*, Vols. 1 and 2. A. Maloine. Paris (1911).

[2] Loewi O. (1921) Uber humorale Ubertragbarkeit des Herznervenwirkung. *Pflugers Arch. 189*, 239-42.

[3] Dale HH. (1935) Pharmacology and nerve-endings. *Proc R Soc Med. 28*, 319-32.

[4] Kandel ER, Schwartz JH, Jessell TM. *Principles of Neural Science*. Publisher: McGraw-Hill Medical; 4 edition (January 5, 2000).

[5] Eccles JC. (1976) From electrical to chemical transmission in the central nervous system. *R. Soc. London Notes and records. 30*, 219-30.

[6] Burnstock G. (1976) Do some nerve cells release more than one transmitter? *Neurosci. 1*, 239-48.

[7] Overstreet LS. (2005) Quantal transmission: not just for neurons. *Trends Neurosci. 28*, 59-62.

[8] Dunant Y, Israel M. (1998) In vitro reconstitution of neurotransmitter release. *Neurochem Res.* 23, 709-18.

[9] Shigeri Y, Seal RP, Shimamoto K. (2004) Molecular pharmacology of glutamate transporters, EAATs and VGLUTs. *Brain Res. Brain Res Rev. 45*, 250-65.

[10] Curtis DR, Johnston GA. (1974) Amino acid transmitters in the mammalian central nervous system. *Ergeb Physiol. 69*, 97-188.

[11] Rogawski MA, Barker JL. *Neurotransmitter actions in the vertebrate nervous system.* Edited by Rogawski MA and Barker JL. Plenum Press New York and London (1985).

[12] Nicoll RA. (1988) The coupling of neurotransmitter receptors to ion channels in the brain. *Science. 241*, 545-51.

[13] Roberts E. (1991) Living systems are tonically inhibited, autonomous optimizers, and disinhibition coupled to variability generation is their major organizing principle: inhibitory command-control at levels of membrane, genome, metabolism, brain, and society. *Neurochem Res. 16*, 409-21.

[14] Curtis DR, Phillis JW, Watkins JC. (1959) Chemical excitation of spinal neurons. *Nature. 183*, 611-2.

[15] Storm-Mathisen J, Leknes AK, Bore AT, Vaaland JL, Edminson P, Haug FS, Ottersen OP. (1983) First visualization of glutamate and GABA in neurones by immunochemistry. *Nature, 301*, 517-20.

[16] Headley PM, Grillner S. (1990) Excitatory amino acids and synaptic transmission: the evidence for a physiological function. *TIPS. 11*, 205-11.

[17] Watkins JC. (2000) l-glutamate as a central neurotransmitter: looking back. *Biochem Soc Trans. 28*, 297-309.

[18] Fonnum F. (1984) Glutamate: a neurotransmitter in mammalian brain. *J Neurochem. 42*, 1-11.

[19] Ribak CE, Seress L. (1983) Five types of basket cell in the hippocampal dentate gyrus: a combined Golgi and electron microscopic study. *J Neurocytol. 12*, 577-97.

[20] Seress L, Ribak CE. (1983) GABAergic cells in the dentate gyrus appear to be local circuit and projection neurons. *Exp Brain Res. 50*, 173-82.

[21] Crawford I, Connor J. (1973) Localization and release of glutamic acid in relation to the hippocampal mossy fiber pathway. *Nature. 244*, 442-3.

[22] Cotman CW, Flatman JA, Ganong AH, Perkins MN. (1986) Effects of excitatory amino acid antagonists on evoked and spontaneous excitatory potentials in guinea-pig hippocampus. *J. Physiol (London). 378*, 403-15.

[23] Lambert JD, Jones RS, Andreasen M, Jensen MS, Heinemann U. (1989) The role of excitatory amino acids in synaptic transmission in the hippocampus. *Comp Biochem Physiol A. 93*, 195-201.

[24] Langdon RB, Johnson JW, Barrionuevo G. (1993) Asynchrony of mossy fibre inputs and excitatory postsynaptic currents in rat hippocampus. *J Physiol. 472*, 157-76.

[25] McBain CJ, Freund TF, Mody I. (1999) Glutamatergic synapses onto hippocampal interneurons: precision timing without lasting plasticity. *Trends Neurosci. 22*, 228-35.

[26] Andersen P, Bliss TV, Lomo T, Olsen LI, Skrede KK. (1969) Lamellar organization of hippocampal excitatory pathways. *Acta Physiol Scand. 76*, 4A-5A.

[27] Amaral DG, Witter MP. (1989) The three-dimensional organization of the hippocampal formation: a review of anatomical data. *Neurosci. 31*, 571-91.

[28] Andersen P, Soleng AF, Raastad M. (2000) The hippocampal lamella hypothesis revisited. *Brain Res. 886*, 165-71.

[29] Hertz L. (2004) Intercellular metabolic compartmentation in the brain: past, present and future. *Neurochem Int. 45*, 285-96.

[30] Kew JN, Kemp JA. (2005) Ionotropic and metabotropic glutamate receptor structure and pharmacology. Psychopharmacology (Berl). 179, 4-29. Erratum in: (2005) *Psychopharmacology (Berl). 182*, 320.

[31] Monaghan D T, Bridges RJ, Cotman C W. (1989) The excitatory amino acid receptors: their classes, pharmacology, and distinct properties in the function of the central nervous system. *Ann. Rev. Pharmacol Toxicol. 29*, 365-402.

[32] Watkins JC, Krogsgaard-Larsen P, Honoré T. (1990) Structure-activity relationships in the development of excitatory amino acid receptor agonists and competitive antagonists. *TIPS. 11*, 25-38.

[33] Fagg GE, Foster AC. (1983) Amino acid neurotransmitters and their pathways in the mammalian central nervous system. *Neurosci. 9*, 701-19.

[34] Balcar VJ, Johnston GA. (1972) The structural specificity of the high affinity uptake of L-glutamate and L-aspartate by rat brain slices. *J Neurochem. 19*, 2657-66.

[35] Davies LP, Johnston GA. (1976) Uptake and release of D- and L-aspartate by rat brain slices. *J Neurochem. 26*, 1007-14.

[36] Attwell D, Barbour B, Szatkowski M. (1993) Nonvesicular release of neurotransmitter. *Neuron. 11*, 401-7.

[37] Burger PM, Mehl E, Cameron PL, Maycox PR, Baumert M, Lottspeich F, De Camilli P, Jahn R. (1989) Synaptic vesicles immunoisolated from rat cerebral cortex contain high levels of glutamate. *Neuron. 3*, 715-20.

[38] Takamori S, Rhee JS, Rosenmund C, Jahn R. (2000) Identification of a vesicular glutamate transporter that defines a glutamatergic phenotype in neurons. *Nature. 407*, 189-94.

[39] Fremeau RT Jr, Voglmaier S, Seal RP, Edwards RH. (2004) VGLUTs define subsets of excitatory neurons and suggest novel roles for glutamate. *Trends Neurosci. 27*, 98-103.

[40] Roberts E, Frankel S. (1950) Aminobutyric acid in brain: its formation from glutamic acid. *J Biol Chem. 187*, 55-63.

[41] Wu jY, Roberts E. (1974) Properties of brain L-glutamate decarboxylase: inhibition studies. *J Neurochem. 23*, 759-67.

[42] Reubi JC, Van Der Berg C, Cuénod M. (1978) Glutamine as precursor for the GABA and glutamate transmitter pools. *Neurosci Letters. 10*, 171-4.

[43] Erlander MG, Tillakaratne NJ, Feldblum S, Patel N, Tobin AJ. (1991) Two genes encode distinct glutamate decarboxylases. *Neuron. 7*, 91-100.

[44] Erlander MG, Tobin AJ. (1991) The structural and functional heterogeneity of glutamic acid decarboxylase: a review. *Neurochem Res. 16*, 215-26.

[45] Kaufman DL, Houser CR, Tobin AJ. (1991) Two forms of the gamma-aminobutyric acid synthetic enzyme glutamate decarboxylase have distinct intraneuronal distributions and cofactor interactions. *J Neurochem. 56*, 720-3.

[46] Miller LP, Walters JR. (1979) Effects of depolarization on cofactor regulation of glutamic acid decarboxylase in substantia nigra synaptosomes. *J Neurochem. 33*, 533-9.

[47] Miller LP, Walters JR, Eng N, Martin DL. (1980) Glutamate holodecarboxylase levels and regulation of GABA synthesis. *Brain Res Bull. 5*, 89-94.

[48] Martin DL, Rimvall K. (1993) Regulation of gamma-aminobutyric acid synthesis in the brain. *J. Neurochem. 60*, 395-407.

[49] Waagepetersen HS, Sonnewald U, Gegelashvili G, Larsson OM, Schousboe A. (2001) Metabolic distinction between vesicular and cytosolic GABA in cultured GABAergic neurons using 13C magnetic resonance spectroscopy. *J Neurosci Res. 63*, 347-55.

[50] Matsumoto RR. (1989) GABA receptors: are cellular differences reflected in function? *Brain Res Rev. 14*, 203-25.

[51] Bowery NG, Hudson AL, Price GW. (1987) GABA-A and GABA-B receptor site distribution in the rat central nervous system. *Neurosci. 20*, 365-33.

[52] Mohler H. (2006) GABA(A) receptor diversity and pharmacology. *Cell Tissue Res. 326*, 505-16.

[53] Sivilotti L, Nistri A. (1991) GABA receptor mechanisms in the central nervous system. *Progress in Neurobiology. 36*, 35-92.

[54] Kornau HC. (2006) GABA(B) receptors and synaptic modulation. *Cell Tissue Res. 326*, 517-33.

[55] Bernath S, Zigmond MJ. (1988) Characterization of [3H] GABA release from striatal slices: evidence for a calcium-independent process via the GABA uptake system. *Neurosci. 27*, 563-70.

[56] Pin JP, Bockaert J. (1989) Two distinct mechanism, differentially affected by excitatory amino acids, trigger GABA release from fetal mouse striatal neurons in primary culture. *J Neurosci. 8*, 648-56.

[57] Iversen LL, Kelly JS. (1975) Uptake and metabolism of gamma-aminobutyric acid by neurones and glial cells. *Biochem Pharmacol. 24*, 933-8.

[58] Radian R, Ottersen OP, Storm-Mathisen J, Castel M, Kanner BI. (1990) Immunocytochemical localization of the GABA transporter in rat brain. *J Neurosci. 10*, 1319-30.

[59] Ribak CE, Tong WM, Brecha NC. (1996) GABA plasma membrane transporters, GAT-1 and GAT-3, display different distributions in the rat hippocampus. *J Comp Neurol. 367*, 595-606.

[60] Sihra TS, Nicholls DG. (1987) 4-Aminobutyrate can be released exocytotically from guinea-pig cerebral cortical synaptosomes. *J Neurochem. 49*, 261-7.

[61] Belhage B, Hansen GH, Schousboe A. (1993) Depolarization by K+ and glutamate activates different neurotransmitter release mechanisms in GABAergic neurons: vesicular versus non-vesicular release of GABA. *Neurosci. 54*, 1019-34.

[62] McIntire SL, Reimer RJ, Schuske K, Edwards RH, Jorgensen EM. (1997) Identification and characterization of the vesicular GABA transporter. *Nature. 389*, 870-6.

[63] Sagne C, El Mestikawy S, Isambert MF, Hamon M, Henry JP, Giros B, Gasnier B. (1997) Cloning of a functional vesicular GABA and glycine transporter by screening of genome databases. *FEBS Lett. 417*, 177-83.

[64] Chaudhry FA, Reimer RJ, Bellocchio EE, Danbolt NC, Osen KK, Edwards RH Storm-Mathisen J. (1998) The vesicular GABA transporter, VGAT, localizes to synaptic vesicles in sets of glycinergic as well as GABAergic neurons. *J Neurosci. 18*, 9733-50.

[65] Iadarola MJ, Gale K. (1981) Cellular compartments of GABA in brain and their relationship to anticonvulsant activity. *Mol Cell Biochem. 39*, 305-29.

[66] Ribak CE, Vaughn JE, Saito K. (1978) Immunocytochemical localization of glutamic acid decarboxylase in neuronal somata following colchicine inhibition of axonal transport. *Brain Res. 140*, 315-32.

[67] Ottersen OP, Storm-Mathisen J. (1984) Glutamate- and GABA-containing neurons in the mouse and rat brain, as demonstrated with a new immunocytochemical technique. *J Comp Neurol. 229*, 374-92.

[68] Hobson JA, McCarley RW, Wyzinski PW. (1975) Sleep cycle oscillation: reciprocal discharge by two brainstem neuronal groups. *Science. 189*, 55-8.

[69] Aston-Jones G, Bloom FE. (1981) Activity of norepinephrine-containing locus coeruleus neurons in behaving rats anticipates fluctuations in the sleep-waking cycle. *J Neurosci. 1*, 876-86.

[70] Somogyi J, Llewellyn-Smith IJ. (2001) Patterns of colocalization of GABA, glutamate and glycine immunoreactivities in terminals that synapse on dendrites of noradrenergic neurons in rat locus coeruleus. *Eur J Neurosci. 14*, 219-28.

[71] Ornung G, Ottersen OP, Cullheim S, Ulfhake B. (1998) Distribution of glutamate-, glycine- and GABA-immunoreactive nerve terminals on dendrites in the cat spinal motor nucleus. *Exp Brain Res. 118*, 517-32.

[72] Somogyi J. (2002) Differences in ratios of GABA, glycine and glutamate immunoreactivities in nerve terminals on rat hindlimb motoneurons: a possible source of post-synaptic variability. *Brain Res Bull. 59*, 151-61.

[73] Kisvarday ZF, Cowey A, Smith AD, Somogyi P. (1989) Interlaminar and lateral excitatory amino acid connections in the striate cortex of monkey. *J Neurosci. 9*, 667-82.

[74] White LE, Hodges HD, Carnes KM, Price JL, Dubinsky JM. (1994) Colocalization of excitatory and inhibitory neurotransmitter markers in striatal projection neurons in the rat. *J Comp Neurol. 339*, 328-40.

[75] Palestini M, Guegan M, Saavedra H, Thomasset M, Batini C. (1993) Glutamate, GABA, calbindin-D28k and parvalbumin immunoreactivity in the pulvinar-lateralis posterior complex of the cat: relation to the projection to the Clare-Bishop area. *Neurosci Lett. 160*, 89-92.

[76] Davanger S, Hjelle OP, Babaie E, Larsson LI, Hougaard D, Storm-Mathisen J, Ottersen OP. (1994) Colocalization of gamma-aminobutyrate and gastrin in the rat antrum: an immunocytochemical and in situ hybridization study. *Gastroenterology. 107*, 137-48.

[77] Sherry DM, Ulshafer RJ. (1992) Neurotransmitter-specific identification and characterization of neurons in the all-cone retina of Anolis carolinensis. II: Glutamate and aspartate. *Vis Neurosci. 9*, 313-23.

[78] Kalloniatis M, Fletcher EL. (1993) Immunocytochemical localization of the amino acid neurotransmitters in the chicken retina. *J Comp Neurol. 336*, 174-93.

[79] Yang CY, Yazulla S. (1994) Glutamate-, GABA-, and GAD-immunoreactivities co-localize in bipolar cells of tiger salamander retina. *Vis Neurosci. 11*, 1193-203.

[80] Batini C, Compoint C, Buisseret-Delmas C, Daniel H, Guegan M. (1992) Cerebellar nuclei and the nucleocortical projections in the rat: retrograde tracing coupled to GABA and glutamate immunohistochemistry. *J Comp Neurol. 315*, 74-84.

[81] Liu CJ, Grandes P, Matute C, Cuenod M, Streit P. (1989) Glutamate-like immunoreactivity revealed in rat olfactory bulb, hippocampus and cerebellum by monoclonal antibody and sensitive staining method. *Histochemistry. 90*, 427-45.

[82] Walberg F, Ottersen OP. (1992) Neuroactive amino acids in the area postrema. An immunocytochemical investigation in rat with some observations in cat and monkey (Macaca fascicularis). *Anat Embryol (Berl). 185*, 529-45.

[83] Marc RE, Liu WL, Kalloniatis M, Raiguel SF, van Haesendonck E. (1990) Patterns of glutamate immunoreactivity in the goldfish retina. *J Neurosci. 10*, 4006-34.

[84] Davanger S, Ottersen OP, Storm-Mathisen J. (1991) Glutamate, GABA, and glycine in the human retina: an immunocytochemical investigation. *J Comp Neurol. 311*, 483-94.

[85] Kalloniatis M, Tomisich G, Marc RE. (1994) Neurochemical signatures revealed by glutamine labeling in the chicken retina. *Vis Neurosci. 11*, 793-804.

[86] Yang CY. (1996) Glutamate immunoreactivity in the tiger salamander retina differentiates between GABA-immunoreactive and glycine-immunoreactive amacrine cells. *J Neurocytol. 25*, 391-403.

[87] Reichenberger I, Straka H, Ottersen OP, Streit P, Gerrits NM, Dieringer N. (1997) Distribution of GABA, glycine, and glutamate immunoreactivities in the vestibular nuclear complex of the frog. *J Comp Neurol. 377*, 149-64.

[88] Quaglino E, Giustetto M, Panzanelli P, Cantino D, Fasolo A, Sassoe-Pognetto M. (1999) Immunocytochemical localization of glutamate and gamma-aminobutyric acid in the accessory olfactory bulb of the rat. *J Comp Neurol. 408*, 61-72.

[89] Llewellyn-Smith IJ, Martin CL, Minson JB. (2002) Glutamate and GABA content of calbindin-immunoreactive nerve terminals in the rat intermediolateral cell column. *Auton Neurosci. 98*, 7-11.

[90] Mosinger JL, Yazulla S, Studholme KM. (1986) GABA-like immunoreactivity in the vertebrate retina: a species comparison. *Exp Eye Res. 42*, 631-44.

[91] Yang CY, Yazulla S. (1988) Localization of putative GABAergic neurons in the larval tiger salamander retina by immunocytochemical and autoradiographic methods. *J Comp Neurol. 277*, 96-108.

[92] Wassle H, Chun MH. (1989) GABA-like immunoreactivity in the cat retina: light microscopy. *J Comp Neurol. 279*, 43-54.

[93] Llewellyn-Smith IJ, Cassam AK, Krenz NR, Krassioukov AV, Weaver LC. (1997) Glutamate- and GABA-immunoreactive synapses on sympathetic preganglionic neurons caudal to a spinal cord transection in rats. *Neurosci. 80*, 1225-35.

Chapter III

GENE EXPRESSION IN THE HIPPOCAMPUS

ABSTRACT

New high throughput screening technologies, gene and protein arrays, allow the detection of thousands of genes and proteins in one experimental run. They hold the promise to unravel the relation between structure and function of a particular tissue, particularly the central nervous system (CNS). These techniques coupled with traditional histological procedures, like immunohistology and *in situ* hybridization, allow to further refine the investigations at the cellular level. Gene profiling and *in situ* hybridization have been applied to map gene expression in regions of the adult CNS, like the hippocampus. Results from these studies reveal a unique pattern of gene expression in the hippocampus, with genes specifically expressed in various hippocampal subfields. Gene profiling of the hippocampus supports the anatomical division of the hippocampus and gives insights into the understanding of the physiopathology of the hippocampus.

INTRODUCTION

Conventional screening strategies, like immunohistology, *in situ* hybridization, reverse transcriptase-polymerase chain reaction (RT-PCR), northern and western blot, are the main protocols used to study gene expression of a particular tissue [1]. These techniques are mainly limited by the few numbers of genes that can be studied in one experimental run. This renders their applications for the understanding of gene-function relationship a labor intensive and random process, involving high throughput screening and trial by chance experimental work. Despite these limitations, these techniques have proven to be successful in identifying genes expressed in various tissues, like the CNS.

The genomes of mouse, human and rat are nearly completely sequenced and available in databases [2-7]. New tools have been developed and optimized to take advantage of this vast amount of information, to study the relationship gene-function. To this aim, DNA array or gene chip technology has been devised to screen thousands of genes in one single experimental run and softwares have been developed to analyze the generated data [8-13]. A DNA array is composed of thousands of genes synthesized or thousands of probes designed to recognize the gene sequences of a particular genome. The probes are attached to a solid surface or chip, allowing the screening of thousands of genes of a particular genome at once. There are two types of DNA array technologies, spotted microarrays, in which the probes are small oligonucleotides or PCR fragments, and oligonucleotides microarrays, corresponding to large sequences of the genes. DNA array allows large scale study of gene expression or gene profiling of various tissues, particularly the CNS, for various species, including mouse, human and rat [14-15].

Molecular Markers of the Hippocampus

Using conventional screening strategies, like immunohistochemistry, *in situ* hybridization, RT-PCR, northern and western blot, several molecular markers of the hippocampus and its subfields have been identified. Some markers, like microtubule-associated protein-2 (Map-2), are expressed in all the hippocampal regions, dentate gyrus (DG) and *Cornu Ammonis* (CA). Map-2 is a marker for mature neurons of the CNS; it is expressed in the nerve cells' dendrites and perikaryon [16]. In the hippocampus, Map-2 is expressed in granule and pyramidal cells [16].

Other markers are expressed in specific hippocampal subfields. In rodents, the subunit 1 of the kainate receptor (KA1), a glutamate receptor, is expressed in dentate granule cells and CA3-CA4 pyramidal cells [17]. Protein kinase C-βII, the transcription factor SCIP, a transcription factor of the POU family involved in glial differentiation [18], and Tyro3, a tyrosine kinase receptor [19], are expressed in CA1 pyramidal cells [20-23]. The transcription factor Py is expressed in CA3-CA4 pyramidal cells [24]. In these studies, the expression of the markers in CA1 and CA3 regions is overlapping in the region known as CA2 [25]. In contrast, some genes are specifically expressed in CA2 region. Neurotrophin 3 (NT-3), a trophic factor of the nerve growth factor family [26], is expressed in dentate granule cells and CA2 pyramidal cells, but not in CA1 and CA3 pyramidal cells [27,28]. Basic fibroblast growth factor (FGF-2) [29-31], adenosine A1 receptor [32], epidermal growth factor-receptor (EGFR) [33], insulin-like growth factor binding protein-4 (IGFBP4) [34] and trek-2 [35] are also specifically expressed in CA2 pyramidal cells. Acetyl cholinesterase is expressed highest in CA2 pyramidal cells [36,37].

These data show that conventional screening strategies have been successfully applied to identify molecular markers of the hippocampus and its sub-regions. Among these markers, some label cells other than granule and pyramidal cells. Py is detected in interneurons throughout the hippocampus, and Py, KA1, SCIP and Tyro3 label cell types outside the hippocampus [20,22-24,38,39].

The region CA2 and CA4 have been originally defined by Lorente de No (1934), based on histological studies [25]. The CA2 region corresponds to the region of the CA subfield between CA1 and CA3. CA2 region has "giant" pyramidal cells, as in CA3, and does not elicit giant thorny excrescence, corresponding to the region of termination of the mossy fibers (MFs) in CA3 region. The MFs are the axons of the dentate granule cells. The CA4 region corresponds to the CA subfield within the *hilus* of the DG [25]. The existence of CA2 region has been the source of debates, as many investigators consider CA2 region as a small transitional zone between CA1 and CA3 regions without real identity; a region where the two classes of pyramidal neurons of CA1 and CA3 mingle [40-46]. On the one hand, molecular studies show that the expression of markers, like KA1, Protein kinase C-βII, SCIP, Tyro3 and Py, is overlapping in CA2 region. This supports the CA subfield as composed primarily of two regions CA1 and CA3. On the other hand, many genes, like NT-3, FGF-2, adenosine A1 receptor, EGFR, IGFBP4 and trek-2, define remarkably a distinct CA2 region. This indicates that in the hippocampus, a discrete CA2 region exists and can be revealed also molecularly. Whether the CA2 region, defined molecularly and by Lorente de No (1934), corresponds to the same boundaries remains to be determined.

GENE PROFILING OF HIPPOCAMPAL SUB-REGIONS

With the advent of genome-scale molecular techniques, it has become possible to profile global gene expression patterns of isolated tissues [13-15]. These techniques, microarrays, serial analysis of gene expression (SAGE), hold great promise for understanding the structure and function-relationship of a particular tissue. They have been applied to profile gene expression of embryonic and adult brains, as well as particular brain areas, like the amygdale and hippocampus [41,47-53]. These studies reveal specific gene expression profiles in embryonic and adult brain tissues.

To further understand the relationship structure-function between neuronal populations of the adult hippocampus, Zhao et al. (2001) and Lein et al. (2004, 2005) performed comparative gene chip analysis on micro-dissected regions of the adult mouse hippocampus [54-56]. The authors dissected, under the microscope, the DG, CA1 and CA3 regions from 10-week-old mice. CA1 was isolated of the hippocampus using the natural division of the hippocampal fissure that separates CA1 from the DG [57]. The top portion of CA region, dissected out from the hippocampus corresponds to approximately CA1. The remainder of CA region, corresponding to approximately CA3, was dissected from the DG, along clearly visible boundaries [54,55]. The authors isolated RNAs from these three dissected areas using standard procedures and processed them for gene expression profiling on gene chips.

This dissection has several limitations for profiling gene expression of hippocampal sub-regions. First, the hippocampal subfields were not dissected according to Lorente de No description of the hippocampus [25]. Particularly, the hippocampal sub-regions CA2 and CA4 were not discriminated from other regions during the dissection. Adjacent regions to the hippocampus, like the subiculum and fimbria/fornix, were also not completely dissected out. Hence, gene chip analysis of the DG, CA1 and CA3 subfields will be contaminated by RNA expressed in CA2 or CA4 regions, but also from areas adjacent to the hippocampus, the subiculum and fimbria/fornix. Particularly, samples from CA1 and CA3 will be contaminated by RNAs from CA2. Samples from the DG will be contaminated by RNAs from CA4, most likely the proximal portion of CA3 and the *hilus*. Samples from CA1 will also be contaminated by RNAs from a residual section of the adjacent subiculum and samples from CA3 by RNA from the adjacent fimbria/fornix region. To overcome this issue, Zhao et al. (2001) and Lein et al. (2004, 2005) performed in parallel to gene chip analysis, studies at the cellular level using techniques, like *in situ* hybridization. For *in situ* hybridization, the investigators used probes generated against candidate genes identified from the gene chip analysis. This strategy allows not only to determine at the cellular level which particular gene is expressed in a given cell types of the hippocampus, but also to validate the data generated from the gene chip analysis [54-56].

Zhao et al. (2001) reported that when comparing any two regions, a substantial number of genes are differentially expressed in the hippocampal sub-regions [54]. Defining strict criteria for gene selection, like a detection sensitivity of 1.5 fold cut-off changes between groups, Zhao et al. (2001) identified a small set of genes, 34 genes, that are expressed highest either in the DG, CA1 or CA3 region. Using *in situ* hybridization, the authors further defined the hippocampal sub-regions and cell types in which the identified genes are expressed. Among them, the gene Purkinje cell protein 4 (*Pcp4*) is highly expressed in dentate granule cells and CA2 pyramidal cells. The gene *Pcp4* is highly expressed in the brain, primarily in cerebellar Purkinje cells. Its product, PEP19, was originally isolated in rat as a cerebellar peptide which expression is increased postnatal period [58]. Nephroblastoma overexpressed (*nov*) gene is highly expressed in CA1 pyramidal cells. *Nov* gene is a member of a family of genes which encodes secreted matrix-associated proteins [59]. Protein kinase C delta (*Prkcd*) gene is highly expressed in CA3 pyramidal cells. Prkcd is a serine/threonine kinase that plays a key role in growth regulation and tissue remodeling [60]. *IGFBP1* is uniquely expressed in dentate granule cells. IGFBPs modulate the effects of insulin-like growth factors (IGFs), major stimulators of vertebrate growth and development. In mammals, IGFBP-1 inhibits the actions of IGF-I [61].

The pattern of gene expression observed with the genes *Pcp4*, *nov* and *prkcd* matches the cytoarchitectural boundaries of the hippocampal subfields, as observed by cresyl violet or fluorescent dye bisbenzimide staining. Cresyl violet is a Nissl stain that is widely used in histology; it colors cell bodies in a brilliant violet. Fluorescent dye bisbenzimide stains nuclei. Standard histological stains, like cresyl violet and fluorescent dye bisbenzimide, delineate the cytoarchitectural boundaries of the hippocampal subfields, with the exception of CA2/CA3 boundary [54]. These results highlight the existence of a pattern of expression of region-specific genes in the adult hippocampus. From these results a genetic map of the hippocampus can be drawn. The dentate granule cells and pyramidal cells of CA2 are defined by expression of *Pcp4*. CA1 pyramidal cells express high levels of *nov* and CA3 pyramidal cells are uniquely defined by expression of *prkcd* [54].

Lein et al. (2005) aimed at further expanding the gene profiling analysis conducted by Zhao et al. (2001), to develop a molecular "atlas" of the hippocampus [55]. Using less stringent analytical criteria and a larger set of data, the authors extended the list of candidate genes predicted to be enriched in each of the dissected hippocampal sub-regions. A methodology for high throughput *in situ* hybridization was devised to examine the expression pattern of over 100 genes predicted to have the highest or lowest expression in one of the sub-regions.

From this analysis, other genes were identified to be enriched in hippocampal sub-regions. Among them, *desmoplakin* is uniquely expressed in dentate granule cells. Desmoplakin is a component of desmosomal tight junctions in peripheral tissues [62]. *Mannosidase 1 alpha* (*Man1a*) is highly enriched in CA1 pyramidal cells. Man1a contributes to proteasomal degradation of misfolded glycoproteins. It belongs to the class I alpha 1,2-

mannosidases, conserved through eukaryotic evolution [63]. *Bcl-2-related ovarian killer* (*bok*) is highly enriched in CA3 pyramidal cells. Bok is a proapoptotic protein; it belongs to the bcl-2 family of proteins that play a key role during apoptosis [64]. *Mini chromosome maintenance deficient 6*, a gene involved in initiation of DNA replication in *C. elegans*, is also uniquely expressed in dentate granule cells relative to pyramidal cells of CA regions. It is also highly expressed in interneurons of the *hilus* and *stratum oriens* of CA regions, and throughout most of the brain. *Calretinin*, a marker for subpopulations of inhibitory neuronal cells in the brain [65,66], is enriched in the DG. *Lipoprotein lipase* (*LPL*), a key enzyme of lipid metabolism that hydrolyses triglycerides, is expressed throughout the pyramidal cell layer with no expression in dentate granule cells. In contrast to calretinin, it is nearly restricted to the hippocampus relative to the rest of the brain. Calcium-binding protein or calbindin D28k (CaBP) is a marker for mature neuronal cells. In the hippocampus, immunohistochemistry reveals that it is expressed in all dentate granule cells and in some, but not all, CA1 and CA2 pyramidal cells [68]. Gene profiling study confirms that CaBP is expressed in dentate granule cells and CA1 pyramidal cells. Neuronal guanine nucleotide exchange factor is also restricted to the DG and CA1.

This study confirms that there are in the adult hippocampus an expression pattern of genes that are region-specific and that this expression pattern concerns a broad range of genes. All combinations of gene patterns have been observed. Some genes are expressed in one region, others in several regions, with all combinations of regions observed, except genes with low expression in CA3 and high levels in all other hippocampal regions. This latter combination was not observed [55]. This study reveals that the adult hippocampus is a mosaic of gene expression. It also reveals differences in gene expression pattern in mice versus other species. Particularly, in mice, *CaBP* is expressed in the dentate granule cells and in CA1 pyramidal cells, whereas in human, it is expressed in the DG, CA1 and CA2 [67]. The gene expression pattern in the hippocampus may underlie functional differences between neuronal populations and species.

In a subsequent study, Lein et al. (2005) aimed at developing a three dimensional map of the hippocampus [56]. The authors focused on genes previously identified as enriched in hippocampal sub-regions, *Pcp4*, *man1a* and *bok*, to map the overall structure of the hippocampus. Results show that the expression of each of these genes is robust throughout the hippocampus within their respective sub-regions. *Pcp4* is expressed in the DG and CA2, *Man1a* in CA1 and *bok* in CA3. It also shows that CA2 as defined by *Pcp4* expression consists of a thin zone between, but non-overlapping with CA1 as defined by Man1a and CA3 as defined by Bok. The CA2 region as defined with *Pcp4*, *man1a* and *bok* expression has a fairly uniform width along almost the entire septotemporal axis of the hippocampus. This study confirms that there are consistent genetic boundaries that mirror cytoarchitectural boundaries in the hippocampus [56].

Taken together, these data show that hippocampal sub-regions CA1, CA2, CA3 and the DG can be differentiated on the basis of specific gene expression (table 1). Hence, the DG, CA1, CA2, and CA3 sub-regions of the hippocampus defined by Lorente de No (1934) have a robust genetic counterpart. In all, hippocampal regions are not only histologically different, but also have different gene expression patterns.

Table 1. Summary of genes expressed in adult hippocampal subfields of rodents

Genes	Hippocampal subfields				Reference #
	DG	CA1	CA2	CA3	
Map-2	+	+	+	+	16
KA1	+			+	17
PKC-βII		+	+/-		20
SCIP		+	+/-		21
Tyro3		+	+/-		23
Py			+/-	+	24
NT-3	+		+		27, 28
FGF-2	+		+		29-31
A A1 R	+		+		32
EGFR	+		+		33
IGFBP4	+		+		34
Trek-2	+		+		35
Pcp4	+		+		54
Nov		+			54
Prkcd				+	54
IGFBP1	+				54
Desmoplakin	+				55
Man1a		+			55
Bok				+	55
Mcmd6	+				55
Calretinin	+				55
LPL		+	+	+	55
CaBP	+	+			55
Ngnef	+	+			55

DG, dentate gyrus; CA, Cornu Ammonis; Map-2, like microtubule-associated protein-2; KA1, kainate receptor; PKC-βII, Protein kinase C-βII; SCIP, a transcription factor of the POU family; Tyro3, a tyrosine kinase receptor; Py, transcription factor; NT-3, neurotrophin 3; FGF-2, basic fibroblast growth factor; A A1 R, adenosine A1 receptor, EGFR, epidermal growth factor-receptor, IGFBP4, insulin-like growth factor binding protein-4; trek-2, a transcription factor; Pcp4, Purkinje cell protein 4; nov, nephroblastoma overexpressed; prkcd, protein kinase C delta; IGFBP1, insulin-like growth factor binding protein-1; Man1a, mannosidase 1 alpha; bok, bcl-2-related ovarian killer; mcmd6, mini chromosome maintenance deficient 6; LPL, lipoprotein lipase; CaBP, calcium-binding protein or calbindin D28k; ngnef; neuronal guanine nucleotide exchange factor.

Further Considerations Defining the CA2 Region

Molecular and gene profiling studies reveal that gene expression pattern delineate the CA region into three subfields, CA1, CA2 and CA3, as reported by Lorente de No (1934). However, it remains to determine whether the molecularly defined CA2 region corresponds to Lorente de No's CA2 region. Lorente de No defined CA2 as a small region between CA1 and CA3, composed of CA3-like pyramidal cells that do not receive MF input from dentate granule cells and lack the specialized postsynaptic "thorny excrescences" characteristic of MF synapses [25].

Lorente de No identified CA2 region by mean of histological staining, cresyl violet and Golgi staining [25]. On the one hand, estimates based on Lorente de No's criteria, reveal discrepancies in the size of CA2 region, ranging from 100 to 200 um width in rats [69-71]. These data reveal the difficulty in defining CA2 histologically. On the other hand, estimates based on gene or protein expression, reveal a CA2 region with a width ranging from 250 to 500 um in rodents [31-33,56]. This reveals the diversity of gene expression and cell types in this area. In support to this latter contention, morphological and genetic observations of CA2 region reveal that there are multiple populations of neurons within CA2. Some neurons in CA2 share morphological characteristics with either CA1 or CA3 pyramidal cells, and there are multiple populations of neurons in CA2 region with different dendritic morphology and axonal projections [70,71]. Timm's staining of granule cell MFs does not end abruptly at the CA3/CA2 boundary, but rather tapers off toward the border of CA2/CA1. This indicates that there is some MF input to the CA2 region [72]. FGF-2 is only expressed in approximately 25% of the neurons of CA2 in rat [31] and very little overlap between the different sub-regions have been reported for this gene [54-56]. In contrast, *Adenosine A1 receptor* gene is expressed in CA2 and the adjacent CA3 region, as defined by Lorente de No [32]. The afferent projections from the hypothalamic projection from the supramamilary nucleus terminate in a zone containing the CA2 region and the adjacent CA3 region [73-75]. The pattern of expression of the *Adenosine A1 receptor* would correspond to this latter region, rather than CA2. This shows that morphological and molecular studies support the existence of CA2 as an entity, but also reveals the diversity of gene expression and cell types in this area.

The existence of CA2 has been the source of debates. Many investigators consider CA2 region as a small transitional zone between CA1 and CA3 without real identity, where the two classes of pyramidal neurons of CA1 and CA3 mingle [72,76-80]. The data presented support the existence of the Lorente de No CA2 region with a real identity, but reveal that the CA2 region is composed of heterogeneous cell types. On the one hand, the boundary between CA1 and CA2 are clearly delineated with cresyl violet staining, but not the boundary between CA2 and CA3 regions [25,76,79,80]. On the other hand, though gene expression pattern confirms the existence of CA2 region, due to cellular heterogeneity in CA2 region, some gene expressed in CA2 are also expressed in adjacent regions and do not delineate CA2. These data highlight the difficulty is defining CA2 region histologically, morphologically and genetically.

In all, genetic analysis supports the existence of CA2 as an individual entity of the CA region. Genetic analysis reveals that the extent of CA2 defined molecularly is broader than that defined by Lorente de No's. The afferent projections from the hypothalamic projection from the supramamilary nucleus terminate in a zone containing the CA2 region and the adjacent CA3 region [73-75]. This shows that genetic analysis may underlie physiological differences between pyramidal cell types and regions in the hippocampus.

Conclusion

The screening of thousands of genes in a single experimental run using DNA array technology has revolutionized genetic studies. Gene profiling complemented with analysis at the cellular level, like *in situ* hybridization and immunohistochemistry, allows the mapping of gene expression in individual cell types. This provides invaluable information for our understanding of the structure and relation structure-function of the tissues, particularly the brain. The hippocampus consists of a series of cytoarchitecturally discrete sub-regions that are discriminated from one another based on morphological, connectivity and electrophysiological properties. Gene profiling combined with studies at the cellular level reveals that hippocampal subfields can also be characterized based on gene expression.

Results from these studies indicate the existence of a pattern of expression of region-specific genes in the adult hippocampus, like the genes *Pcp4*, *nov* and *prkcd*. From these results, a genetic map of the hippocampus can be drawn. Particularly, these data confirm and support the existence of CA2 region as an individual entity of the hippocampus. It further reveals that the CA2 region is heterogeneous, with multiple neuronal subtypes and that the extent of CA2 defined molecularly is broader than that defined by Lorente de No's. These particularities may reflect physiological differences between pyramidal cells within the CA sub-regions, particularly CA2.

Further studies will aim at unraveling the relationship structure-function in the hippocampus. The recent publication of a genome-wide atlas of gene expression of the adult mouse brain will extend our knowledge of the understanding of the relation structure function to other areas of the brain [81-83].

References

[1] Sambrook J, Russell DW. *Molecular Cloning: A Laboratory Manual.* Publisher: Cold Spring Harbor Laboratory Press; 3rd Labmn edition (January 15, 2001).

[2] Venter JC, Adams MD, Myers EW, Li PW, Mural RJ et al. (2001) The sequence of the human genome. *Science. 291*, 1304-51. Erratum in: (2001) *Science. 292*, 1838.

[3] International Human Genome Sequencing Consortium. (2001) Initial sequencing and analysis of the human genome. Nature. 409, 860-921. Erratum in: (2001) *Nature 412*, 565. (2001) Nature. 411, 720.

[4] International Human Genome Mapping Consortium. (2001) A physical map of the human genome. *Nature. 409*, 934-41.

[5] Li S, Cutler G, Liu JJ, Hoey T, Chen L, Schultz PG, Liao J, Ling XB. (2003) A comparative analysis of HGSC and Celera human genome assemblies and gene sets. *Bioinformatics. 19*, 1597-605.

[6] Mouse Genome Sequencing Consortium. (2002) Initial sequencing and comparative analysis of the mouse genome. *Nature. 420*, 520-62.

[7] Rat Genome Sequencing Project Consortium. (2004) Genome sequence of the Brown Norway rat yields insights into mammalian evolution. *Nature. 428*, 493-521.

[8] Fodor SP, Rava RP, Huang XC, Pease AC, Holmes CP, Adams CL. (1993) Multiplexed biochemical assays with biological chips. *Nature. 364*, 555-6.

[9] Schena M, Shalon D, Davis RW, Brown PO. (1995) Quantitative monitoring of gene expression patterns with a complementary DNA microarray. *Science. 270*, 467-70.

[10] Chee M, Yang R, Hubbell E, Berno A, Huang XC, Stern D, Winkler J, Lockhart DJ, Morris MS, Fodor SP. (1996) Accessing genetic information with high-density DNA arrays. *Science. 274*, 610-4.

[11] Lockhart DJ, Dong H, Byrne MC, Follettie MT, Gallo MV, Chee MS, Mittmann M, Wang C, Kobayashi M, Horton H, Brown EL. (1996) Expression monitoring by hybridization to high-density oligonucleotide arrays. *Nat Biotechnol. 14*, 1675-80.

[12] Zapala MA, Lockhart DJ, Pankratz DG, Garcia AJ, Barlow C, Lockhart DJ. (2002) Software and methods for oligonucleotide and cDNA array data analysis. *Genome Biol. 3*, SOFTWARE0001.

[13] Aimone JB, Gage FH. (2004) Unbiased characterization of high-density oligonucleotide microarrays using probe-level statistics. *J Neurosci Methods. 135*, 27-33.

[14] Lockhart DJ, Winzeler EA. (2000) Genomics, gene expression and DNA arrays. *Nature. 405*, 827-36.

[15] Lockhart DJ, Barlow C. (2001) Expressing what's on your mind: DNA arrays and the brain. *Nat Rev Neurosci. 2*, 63-8.

[16] Bernhardt R, Matus A. (1984) Light and electron microscopic studies of the distribution of microtubule-associated protein 2 in rat brain: a difference between dendritic and axonal cytoskeletons. *J Comp Neurol. 226*, 203-21.

[17] Wisden W, Seeburg PH. (1993) A complex mosaic of high-affinity kainate receptors in rat brain. *J Neurosci. 13*, 3582-98.

[18] Lemke G, Kuhn R, Monuki ES, Weinmaster G. (1991) Expression and activity of the transcription factor SCIP during glial differentiation and myelination. *Ann N Y Acad Sci. 633*, 189-95.

[19] Lemke G, Lu Q. (2003) Macrophage regulation by Tyro 3 family receptors. *Curr Opin Immunol. 15*, 31-6.

[20] Weeber EJ, Atkins CM, Selcher JC, Varga AW, Mirnikjoo B, Paylor R, Leitges M, Sweatt JD. (2000) A role for the beta isoform of protein kinase C in fear conditioning. *J Neurosci. 20*, 5906-14.

[21] Frantz GD, Bohner AP, Akers RM, McConnell SK. (1994) Regulation of the POU domain gene SCIP during cerebral cortical development. *J Neurosci. 14*, 4724-85.

[22] Grove EA, Tole S. (1999) Patterning events and specification signals in the developing hippocampus. *Cereb Cortex. 9*, 551-61.

[23] Lai C, Gore M, Lemke G. (1994) Structure, expression, and activity of Tyro 3, a neural adhesion-related receptor tyrosine kinase. *Oncogene. 9*, 2567-78.

[24] Woodhams PL, Webb M, Atkinson DJ, Seeley PJ. (1989) A monoclonal antibody, Py, distinguishes different classes of hippocampal neurons. *J Neurosci. 9*, 2170-81.

[25] Lorente de No R. (1934) Studies on the structure of the cerebral cortex. II. Continuation of the study of the ammonic system. *J Psychol Neurol (Lpz). 46*, 113-77.

[26] Ernfors P, Ibanez CF, Ebendal T, Olson L, Persson H. (1990) Molecular cloning and neurotrophic activities of a protein with structural similarities to nerve growth factor: developmental and topographical expression in the brain. *Proc Natl Acad Sci U S A. 87*, 5454-8.

[27] Friedman WJ, Ernfors P, Persson H. (1991) Transient and persistent expression of NT-3/HDNF mRNA in the rat brain during postnatal development. *J Neurosci. 11*, 1577-84.

[28] Vigers AJ, Baquet ZC, Jones KR. (2000) Expression of neurotrophin-3 in the mouse forebrain: insights from a targeted LacZ reporter. *J Comp Neurol. 416*, 398-415.

[29] Eckenstein FP, Kuzis K, Nishi R, Woodward WR, Meshul C, Sherman L, Ciment G. (1994) Cellular distribution, subcellular localization and possible functions of basic and acidic fibroblast growth factors. *Biochem Pharmacol. 47*, 103-10.

[30] Gomez-Pinilla F, Lee JW, Cotman CW. (1994) Distribution of basic fibroblast growth factor in the developing rat brain. *Neurosci. 61*, 911-23.

[31] Williams TE, Meshul CK, Cherry NJ, Tiffany NM, Eckenstein FP, Woodward WR. (1996) Characterization and distribution of basic fibroblast growth factor-containing cells in the rat hippocampus. *J Comp Neurol. 370*, 147-58.

[32] Ochiishi T, Saitoh Y, Yukawa A, Saji M, Ren Y, Shirao T, Miyamoto H, Nakata H, Sekino Y. (1999) High level of adenosine A1 receptor-like immunoreactivity in the CA2/CA3a region of the adult rat hippocampus. *Neurosci. 93*, 955-67.

[33] Tucker MS, Khan I, Fuchs-Young R, Price S, Steininger TL, Greene G, Wainer BH, Rosner MR. (1993) Localization of immunoreactive epidermal growth factor receptor in neonatal and adult rat hippocampus. *Brain Res. 631*, 65-71.

[34] Stenvers KL, Zimmermann EM, Gallagher M, Lund PK. (1994) Expression of insulin-like growth factor binding protein-4 and -5 mRNAs in adult rat forebrain. *J Comp Neurol. 339*, 91-105.

[35] Gu W, Schlichthorl G, Hirsch JR, Engels H, Karschin C, Karschin A, Derst C, Steinlein OK, Daut J. (2002) Expression pattern and functional characteristics of two novel splice variants of the two-pore-domain potassium channel TREK-2. *J Physiol. 539*, 657-68.

[36] Mellgren SI, Harkmark W, Srebro B. (1977) Some enzyme histochemical characteristics of the human hippocampus. *Cell Tissue Res. 181*, 459-71.

[37] Bakst I, Amaral DG. (1984) The distribution of acetylcholinesterase in the hippocampal formation of the monkey. *J Comp Neurol. 225*, 344-71.

[38] He X, Treacy MN, Simmons DM, Ingraham HA, Swanson LW, Rosenfeld MG. (1989) Expression of a large family of POU-domain regulatory genes in mammalian brain development. Nature. 340, 35-41. Erratum in: (1989) *Nature. 340*, 662.

[39] Alvarez-Bolado G, Rosenfeld MG, Swanson LW. (1995) Model of forebrain regionalization based on spatiotemporal patterns of POU-III homeobox gene expression, birthdates, and morphological features. *J Comp Neurol. 355*, 237-95.

[40] Blackstad TW. (1956) Commissural connections of the hippocampal region in the rat, with special reference to their mode of termination. *J Comp Neurol. 105*, 417-537.

[41] Tole S, Christian C, Grove EA. (1977) Early specification and autonomous development of cortical fields in the mouse hippocampus. *Development. 124*, 4959-70.

[42] Swanson LW, Cowan WM. (1977) An autoradiographic study of the organization of the efferent connections of the hippocampal formation in the rat. *J Comp Neurol. 172*, 49-84.

[43] Swanson LW, Wyss JM, Cowan WM. (1978) An autoradiographic study of the organization of intrahippocampal association pathways in the rat. *J Comp Neurol. 181*, 681-715.

[44] Zimmer J, Haug FM. (1978) Laminar differentiation of the hippocampus, fascia dentata and subiculum in developing rats, observed with the Timm sulphide silver method. *J Comp Neurol. 179*, 581-617

[45] Gaarskjaer FB. (1986) The organization and development of the hippocampal mossy fiber system. *Brain Res. 396*, 335-57.

[46] Woodhams PL, Celio MR, Ulfig N, Witter MP. (1993) Morphological and functional correlates of borders in the entorhinal cortex and hippocampus. *Hippocampus. 3*, 303-11.

[47] Luo L, Salunga RC, Guo H, Bittner A, Joy KC, Galindo JE, Xiao H, Rogers KE, Wan JS, Jackson MR, Erlander MG. (1999) Gene expression profiles of laser-captured adjacent neuronal subtypes. Nat Med. 5, 117-22. Erratum in: (1999) *Nat Med. 5*, 355.

[48] Sandberg R, Yasuda R, Pankratz DG, Carter TA, Del Rio JA, Wodicka L, Mayford M, Lockhart DJ, Barlow C. (2000) Regional and strain-specific gene expression mapping in the adult mouse brain. *Proc Natl Acad Sci U S A. 97*, 11038-43.

[49] Zirlinger M, Kreiman G, Anderson DJ. (2001) Amygdala-enriched genes identified by microarray technology are restricted to specific amygdaloid subnuclei. *Proc Natl Acad Sci U S A. 98*, 5270-5.

[50] Datson NA, van der Perk J, de Kloet ER, Vreugdenhil E. (2001) Expression profile of 30,000 genes in rat hippocampus using SAGE. *Hippocampus. 11*, 430-44.

[51] Mody M, Cao Y, Cui Z, Tay KY, Shyong A, Shimizu E, Pham K, Schultz P, Welsh D, Tsien JZ. (2001) Genome-wide gene expression profiles of the developing mouse hippocampus. *Proc Natl Acad Sci U S A. 98*, 8862-7.

[52] Zapala MA, Hovatta I, Ellison JA, Wodicka L, Del Rio JA, Tennant R, Tynan W, Broide RS, Helton R, Stoveken BS, Winrow C, Lockhart DJ, Reilly JF, Young WG, Bloom FE, Lockhart DJ, Barlow C. (2005) Adult mouse brain gene expression patterns bear an embryologic imprint. *Proc Natl Acad Sci U S A. 102*, 10357-62.

[53] Korostynski M, Kaminska-Chowaniec D, Piechota M, Przewlocki R. (2006) Gene expression profiling in the striatum of inbred mouse strains with distinct opioid-related phenotypes. *BMC Genomics. 7*, 146.

[54] Zhao X, Lein ES, He A, Smith SC, Aston C, Gage FH. (2001) Transcriptional profiling reveals strict boundaries between hippocampal subregions. *J Comp Neurol. 441*, 187-96.

[55] Lein ES, Zhao X, Gage FH. (2004) Defining a molecular atlas of the hippocampus using DNA microarrays and high-throughput in situ hybridization. *J Neurosci. 24*, 3879-89.

[56] Lein ES, Callaway EM, Albright TD, Gage FH. (2005) Redefining the boundaries of the hippocampal CA2 subfield in the mouse using gene expression and 3-dimensional reconstruction. *J Comp Neurol. 485*, 1-10.

[57] Taupin P, Zini S, Cesselin F, Ben-Ari Y, Roisin MP. (1994) Subcellular fractionation on Percoll gradient of mossy fiber synaptosomes: morphological and biochemical characterization in control and degranulated rat hippocampus. *J Neurochem. 62*, 1586-95.

[58] Sangameswaran L, Hempstead J, Morgan JI. (1989) Molecular cloning of a neuron-specific transcript and its regulation during normal and aberrant cerebellar development. *Proc Natl Acad Sci U S A. 86*, 5651-5.

[59] Perbal B. NOV (nephroblastoma overexpressed) and the CCN family of genes: structural and functional issues. (2001) *Mol Pathol. 54*, 57-79.

[60] Steinberg SF. (2004) Distinctive activation mechanisms and functions for protein kinase Cdelta. *Biochem J. 384*, 449-59.

[61] Mounier C, Posner BI. (2006) Transcriptional regulation by insulin: from the receptor to the gene. *Can J Physiol Pharmacol. 84*, 713-24.

[62] Kowalczyk AP, Borgwardt JE, Green KJ. (1996) Analysis of desmosomal cadherin-adhesive function and stoichiometry of desmosomal cadherin-plakoglobin complexes. *J Invest Dermatol. 107*, 293-300.

[63] Herscovics A. (2001) Structure and function of Class I alpha 1,2-mannosidases involved in glycoprotein synthesis and endoplasmic reticulum quality control. *Biochimie. 83*, 757-62.

[64] Hsu SY, Hsueh AJ. (2000) Tissue-specific Bcl-2 protein partners in apoptosis: An ovarian paradigm. *Physiol Rev. 80*, 593-614.

[65] Miettinen R, Gulyas AI, Baimbridge KG, Jacobowitz DM, Freund TF. (1992) Calretinin is present in non-pyramidal cells of the rat hippocampus--II. Co-existence with other calcium binding proteins and GABA. *Neurosci. 48*, 29-43.

[66] Gonchar Y, Burkhalter A. (2003) Distinct GABAergic targets of feedforward and feedback connections between lower and higher areas of rat visual cortex. *J Neurosci. 23*, 10904-12.

[67] Sloviter RS. (1989) Calcium-binding protein (calbindin-D28k) and parvalbumin immunocytochemistry: localization in the rat hippocampus with specific reference to the selective vulnerability of hippocampal neurons to seizure activity. *J Comp Neurol. 280*, 183-96.

[68] Maguire-Zeiss KA, Li ZW, Shimoda LM, Hamill RW. (1995) Calbindin D28k mRNA in hippocampus, superior temporal gyrus and cerebellum: comparison between control and Alzheimer disease subjects. *Brain Res. Mol Brain Res. 30*, 362-6.

[69] Swanson LW, Wyss JM, Cowan WM. (1978) An autoradiographic study of the organization of intrahippocampal association pathways in the rat. *J Comp Neurol. 181*. 681-715.

[70] Ishizuka N, Cowan WM, Amaral DG. (1995) A quantitative analysis of the dendritic organization of pyramidal cells in the rat hippocampus. *J Comp Neurol. 362*, 17-45.

[71] Tamamaki N, Abe K, Nojyo Y. (1988) Three-dimensional analysis of the whole axonal arbors originating from single CA2 pyramidal neurons in the rat hippocampus with the aid of a computer graphic technique. *Brain Res. 452*, 255-72.

[72] Gaarskjaer FB. (1986) The organization and development of the hippocampal mossy fiber system. *Brain Res. 396*, 335-57.

[73] Segal M. (1979) A potent inhibitory monosynaptic hypothalamo-hippocampal connection. *Brain Res. 162*, 137-41.

[74] Wyss JM, Swanson LW, Cowan WM. (1979) Evidence for an input to the molecular layer and the stratum granulosum of the dentate gyrus from the supramammillary region of the hypothalamus. *Anat Embryol (Berl). 156*, 165-76.

[75] Stanfield BB, Cowan WM. (1984) An EM autoradiographic study of the hypothalamo-hippocampal projection. *Brain Res. 309*, 299-307.

[76] Blackstad TW. (1956) Commissural connections of the hippocampal region in the rat, with special reference to their mode of termination. *J Comp Neurol. 105*, 417-537.

[77] Tole S, Christian C, Grove EA. (1977) Early specification and autonomous development of cortical fields in the mouse hippocampus. *Development. 124*, 4959-70.

[78] Swanson LW, Cowan WM. (1977) An autoradiographic study of the organization of the efferent connections of the hippocampal formation in the rat. *J Comp Neurol. 172*, 49-84.

[79] Zimmer J, Haug FM. (1978) Laminar differentiation of the hippocampus, fascia dentata and subiculum in developing rats, observed with the Timm sulphide silver method. *J Comp Neurol. 179*, 581-617

[80] Woodhams PL, Celio MR, Ulfig N, Witter MP. (1993) Morphological and functional correlates of borders in the entorhinal cortex and hippocampus. *Hippocampus. 3*, 303-11.

[81] Brill D. (2006) Mouse brain map is complete. *Nature. 443*, 380-1.

[82] Lein ES, Hawrylycz MJ, Ao N, Ayres M, Bensinger A, et al. (2007) Genome-wide atlas of gene expression in the adult mouse brain. *Nature. 445*, 168-76.

[83] Jessberger S, Gage FH. (2007) ZOOMING IN: a new high-resolution gene expression atlas of the brain. *Mol Syst Biol. 3*, 75.

Chapter IV

GRANULE CELLS AND MOSSY FIBERS

ABSTRACT

The granule cells are the nerve cells of the main layer of the hippocampal dentate gyrus (DG), the granule cell layer or *stratum granulosum*. The granule cells are glutamatergic excitatory, component of the hippocampal tri-synaptic circuit. Their axons, the mossy fibers (MFs), project to the *Cornu Ammonis* (CA) region CA3 and establish synaptic contacts with dendritic spines of the pyramidal cells, in a region referred to as the *stratum lucidum*. On the histological level, the synapses MF-CA3 pyramidal cells are characterized by their large size, up to 10 μm diameter, high synaptic density and complex morphology, with dendritic spines invaginated in the boutons. On the biochemical level, the MF synapses are enriched in multiple chemical substances. The MF synapses are enriched in dynorphin and zinc. They also contain other peptides and proteins, including enkephalins and trophic factors. More recently, γ-aminobutyric acid (GABA)-immunoreactivity was identified in the synapses MF-CA3 pyramidal cells. The existence of an inhibitory amino acid transmitter in an excitatory glutamatergic raises the question of the role of GABA in MF terminals (MFTs). The synapse MF-CA3 pyramidal cells can be isolated from other cellular structures, by subcellular fractionation. MF synaptosomes provide a model of choice to study the MF-CA3 pyramidal cell synapses *ex vivo*.

INTRODUCTION

The granule cells are the main cell type of the principal layer of the DG, the granule cell layer or *stratum granulosum*. Their axons, the MFs, originate from the basal level of the soma of the granule cells and cross the *hilus* to reach the pyramidal cells of the CA3 region. They have a mean diameter of 0.5 μm and are unmyelinated [1,2]. They receive their main afferences from the pyramidal cells of the layer II of the entorhinal cortex [3]. The MFs establish synaptic contacts with CA3 pyramidal cells, primarily at the level of the dendritic spines, in a region known as the *stratum lucidum* [4]. The MFs establish synaptic contacts with inhibitory interneurons. These latter are the main targets of the MFs. The MFs establish synaptic contacts with inhibitory interneurons of the CA3 region and polymorphic layer of the hippocampus, characterized by the presence at regular interval (140 um) of synapses, known as synapses "en passant" [6]. Upon staining with Golgi stain, the axons of the granule cells have a mossy appearance, at the origin of the name "mossy fibers" that have been given to them [7]. The synapses MF-CA3 pyramidal cells elicit characteristic histological, biochemical and physiopathological features.

The Mossy Fiber-CA3 Pyramidal Cell Synapses

Histology of Mossy Fiber Terminals

The synapses MF-CA3 pyramidal cells or MF terminals (MFTs) are characterized by their large size, complex morphology and synaptic vesicles density. The mean diameter of synapses in the nervous system is in the range of 1 μm, including the synapses, known as synapses "en passant" between MFs and interneurons [8]. In contrast, the synapses MF-CA3 pyramidal cells (MFTs) have an average diameter of 3 - 5 μm and can reach up to 10 μm diameter [9,10]. MFTs have a complex morphology, with multiple invaginations. They contact one or several dendritic spines of CA3 pyramidal cells that are invaginated within the terminals. They establish both symmetrical and asymmetrical contacts with the post-synaptic regions of the dendritic spines [11]. Asymmetrical synapses are histological criteria indicative of excitatory synapses, whereas symmetrical contacts are indicative of inhibitory synapses. The MFTs contain millions of synaptic vesicles, some of which are core electron dense. Core electron dense synaptic vesicles mostly contain neuropeptides. The MFTs are also characterized by rows of *puncta adherens* [12]. Puncta adherens are cell junctions, with enriched levels of adhesion molecules, like cadherins. In all, the synapses MF-CA3 pyramidal cells elicit unique morphological features that differentiate them from most other synapses of the nervous system. The MFTs are estimated in the mice, at less than 1% of the total number of ending nerves of the hippocampus [13].

Isolation and Purification of Mossy Fiber Terminals: Mossy Fiber Synaptosomes

Synaptosomes are "pinched-off" nerve terminals [14]. Upon homogenization of brain tissues, the synapses are dissociated from the rest of the tissues and formed closed spherical-like particles, named synaptosomes (figure 1). Synaptosomes were first reported by De Robertis et al., in 1961, and Gray and Whittaker, in 1962 [15,16]. The authors studied, by electron microscopy, fractions obtained from brain homogenates, after subcellular fractionation on sucrose gradients. They reported structures of 0.5 μm average diameter, containing mitochondria, synaptic vesicles and postsynaptic densities. They identified these structures as corresponding to the presynaptic ending nerves. Most of the isolated presynaptic terminals present residual components of the postsynaptic membrane [15,16]. They named these structures synaptoneurosomes or synaptosomes. Since then, synaptosomes have been isolated from various brain areas and species using various protocols. Synaptosomes can be isolated and purified using buoyant density by subcellular fractionation, on sucrose, Ficoll and Percoll gradients [17-19]. Among other advantages, the use of Percoll gradients allows a faster purification of synaptosomes in isoosmotic condition, yielding to a more efficient recovery of synaptosomes with a better survival [19]. Synaptosomes have also been successfully isolated and purified by immunoaffinity and fluorescence activated cell sorting [20-25]. Synaptosome preparations have proven their relevance for studying the physiopathology and pharmacology of ending nerves *ex vivo* [26-29].

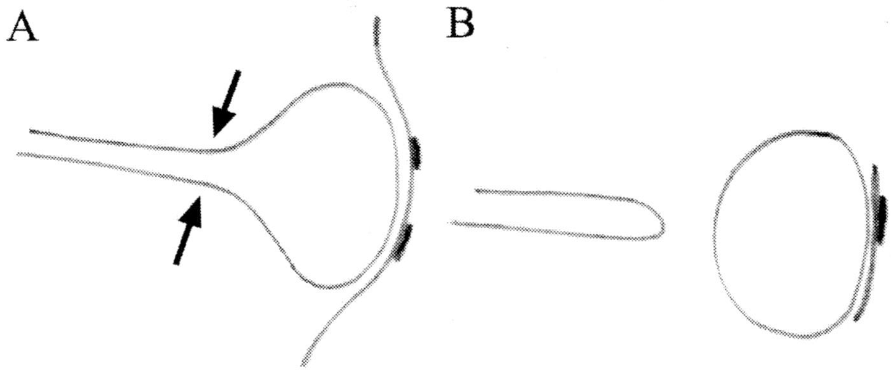

Figure 1. Schematic of "pinched-off" nerve terminals. Synaptosomes are "pinched-off" nerve terminals. Upon homogenization of brain tissues, the synapses are dissociated from the rest of the tissues (A) and formed closed spherical-like particles, named synaptosomes (B). Synaptosomes contain mitochondria, synaptic vesicles and post-synaptic densities.

The large size of the MF-CA3 pyramidal cell synapses allows their isolation from other cellular structures including other nerve terminals, by subcellular fractionation. Several studies have reported the successful isolation and purification of mossy fiber synaptosomes (MFSs) on sucrose-Ficoll and Percoll gradients, from adult rat hippocampus [30-32]. MFSs isolated on Percoll gradients elicit the same features as the MFTs with respect to their morphology; they have a large size, which average 3 μm, as opposed to an average size of 0.5-0.7 μm for other hippocampal synaptosomes (also referred as "small" synaptosomes). They have a complex morphology, with dendritic spines invaginated in the boutons. They also have a high synaptic vesicles density, with some of the synaptic vesicles with core electron dense. Symmetrical and asymmetrical synaptic densities can be observed, together with residual portion of postsynaptic membranes (figure 2) [32]. Dendritic spines invaginated in the MF synaptosomes contain mRNAs. MFS preparations have been successful in identifying RNAs contained in spines [33,34]. In all, MFS preparations provide a model of choice to study the MF-CA3 pyramidal cell synapses *ex vivo*.

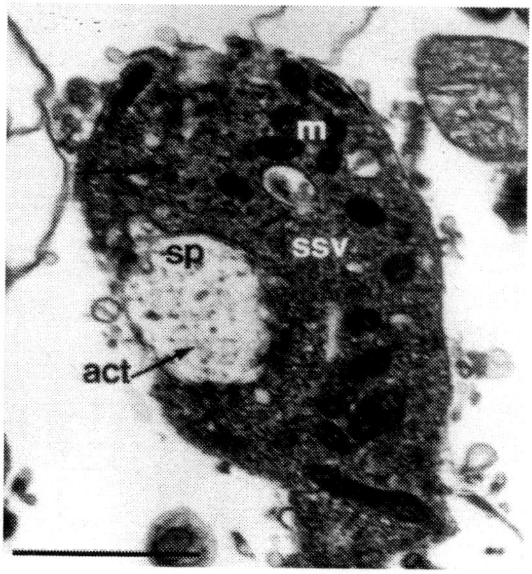

Figure 2. Electron micrograph of a mossy fiber synaptosome. Rat hippocampal mossy fiber synaptosome (MFS) isolated and purified by subcellular fractionation, on Percoll gradients. The granule cells are the nerve cells of the principal layer of the hippocampal dentate gyrus, the granule cell layer. Their axons, the mossy fibers (MFs), project to the region *Cornu Ammonis* (CA) region CA3 of the hippocampus and establish synaptic contact with the dendritic spines of pyramidal cells. The synapses MF-CA3 pyramidal cells elicit unique histological features. The MF synapses have a large size, up to 10 μm diameter, with complex morphology. They contain high synaptic vesicle densities, with core dense synaptic vesicles. The dendritic spines of the pyramidal cells are invaginated in the MF pre-synaptic terminals or boutons. The large size of MF terminals (MFTs) allows their isolation from other cellular structures including other nerve terminals, by subcellular fractionation. Protocols have been devised to isolate and purify MFSs, on Percoll gradients [32]. MFSs isolated on Percoll gradients elicit the same features as the MFTs with respect to their morphology. They have a large size, a complex morphology, with dendritic spines (sp) invaginated in the boutons. They contain a high synaptic vesicles density, with small synaptic vesicles (ssv) and synaptic vesicles with core electron dense. Mitochondria (m) and actin filaments (act) can be observed within the MFTs and dendritic spines, respectively. Scale bar 1 μm.

Biochemistry of Granule Cells and Mossy Fibers

Granule Cells are Glutamatergic Excitatory Nerve Cells

Glutamate (L-glutamic acid, Glu) is the main excitatory neurotransmitter of the nervous system [35,36]. In the hippocampus, Glu is the main excitatory neurotransmitter of the granule and pyramidal cells [37]. Glu was reported for the first time to be neurotransmitter of the granule cells by Crawford and Connor (1973) [38]. Crawford and Connor (1973) made the hypothesis that repetitive stimulations of the MFs produce the accumulation in the CA3 area of Glu, a depolarizing substance. They confirmed their hypothesis by showing that in cat: 1) the concentration of endogenous Glu and glutamine is higher in the CA3 region that contain the MF ending nerves than in the CA1 area, whereas the 5 other amino acids measured, aspartate (L-aspartic acid, Asp), threonine, serine, alanine and glycine show the same distribution, 2) the activity of the biosynthesis enzyme for Glu, the Glu dehydrogenase, is twice more elevated in the region of the MFs than in CA1, and 3) entorhinal stimulation increases significantly the level of Glu released *in vivo* [38]. These results support the role of Glu as a neurotransmitter at the synapse MF-CA3 pyramidal cells.

The role of Glu as the principal neurotransmitter of the synapse MF-CA3 pyramidal cells was subsequently confirmed by other studies. Among them, Storm-Mathisen et al. (1983) reported the presence of Glu in the MF ending nerves by immunohistochemistry in rat [39]. The excitatory postsynaptic potential evoked at the synapse MF-CA3 pyramidal cells is blocked by antagonists of Glu receptors (GluRs), like L-AP4, CNQX [40-42]. Depolarizing concentration of potassium (30-50 mM) evoke the release of Glu, in calcium-dependent manner, from fractions enriched in MFSs of rat hippocampus [31]. In these preparations, the release of Glu is more substantial and significantly more dependent of calcium than the release of aspartate. The low dependence of calcium for the release of Asp suggests that Glu, but not Asp, is the neurotransmitter at the MF synapse. High affinity binding sites for the Glu agonist kainic acid are primarily detected in the *stratum lucidum* and DG of the hippocampus [43-46]. In the *stratum lucidum*, the region of termination of the MFs, excitatory amino acid binding sites are localized in the MF ending nerves [47]. Subcellular fractionation studies have confirmed the presynaptic localization of Glu binding sites and receptors [48]. The metabotropic receptor of Glu is essentially synthesized by the granule cells of the DG and pyramidal cells of the CA2-CA3 region, as shown by *in situ hybridization* [49]. In all, Glu is the main excitatory amino acid at the synapse MF-CA3 pyramidal cells.

Endogenous Opioid Peptides are Enriched in Granule Cells and Mossy Fibers

Opioid peptides, endorphins, enkephalins and dynorphins, are substances naturally present in the organism, particularly the brain [50]. They act through specific receptors. There are three major types of opioid receptors, classified based on their endogenous ligands or agonists: μ(mu)-opioid receptor (agonist: morphine), δ(delta)-opioid receptor (agonist: enkephalin) and κ(kappa)-opioid receptor (agonists: ketocyclazocine, dynorphin) [51]. Opioid peptides, endorphins, enkephalins and dynorphins, derive by post-translational maturation from distinct precursor proteins, prepro-opiomelanocortin (POMC), preproenkephalin and preprodynorphin, respectively [52]. Post-translational maturation of precursor of opioid peptides occurs primarily by proteolysis at basic amino acids [53]. These precursors are encoded by three different genes that share common sequences. Enkephalins have been first reported in the hippocampus by Sar et al. (1978) and Weber et al. (1982) [54,55]. These peptides are localized in the nerve endings [56] and cell bodies [57]. The hippocampus of rat contains higher concentration of dynorphins, particularly the maturation product dynorphin A (1-17), than enkephalin [58].

In 1983, McGinty performed a comparative study of the distribution of dynorphins and enkephalins in the adult rat hippocampus by immunohistochemistry [59]. McGinty (1983) showed that, in the hippocampus, immunoreactivity to an anti-serum against dynorphin A (1-17) is only detected in granule cells and MFs, whereas immunoreactivity to an antiserum against enkephalins is detected in the perforant path, granule cells and MFs. This shows that granule cells and MFs are enriched in dynorphins and contain enkephalins [59]. Granule cells contain other peptides derived from the prodynorphin precursor, like dynorphin B [60], l'alpha neo-endorphin [57] and dynorphin A (1-8) [58]. Electron microscopy analysis reveals that not all the MF ending nerves contain dynorphins [61]. Radio-immunoassays of subcellular fractions confirm the immunohistological localization of opioid peptides in the hippocampus. Dosage of dynorphin B and other products of maturation of the prodynorphin gene, from subcellular fraction of adult rat hippocampus, reveal that dynorphin-immunoreactivity is stronger in fractions enriched in MF synaptosomes than in fractions enriched in other hippocampal synaptosomes or "small" synaptosomes [30,32]. In all, dynorphins are specifically enriched in granule cells and MFs. They are considered markers for granule cells and MFTs.

The presence of dynorphins in granule cells and MFTs raises the question of their involvement in the synapse MF-CA3 pyramidal cells. Dynorphins are released from hippocampal slices, following stimulation of afferent fibers of granule cells [62] and depolarization evoked by potassium in a calcium-dependent manner [58]. Dynorphins are also released from fraction enriched in hippocampal MFSs [30,31,63]. Opioid receptors have been reported in the hippocampus [64]. Weisskopf et al. (1983) reported that auto-receptor kappa are localized presynaptically in MFTs and may be at the origin of the release of dynorphins by the nerve endings [65]. Opioid peptides have excitatory activity on neurons of the hippocampus; these effects are due to a reduction of γ-aminobutyric acid (GABA) inhibition (desinhibition) between interneurons and pyramidal cells [66]. Synaptic release of dynorphin inhibits the induction of long-term potentiation (LTP), at synapse MF-CA3 pyramidal cells [65]. Dynorphins also inhibit the induction of LTP of the synapse perforant path-dentate granule cells. This suggests that dynorphin may act as an inhibitory retrograde neurotransmitter [62]. LTP is a long lasting increase of synaptic efficacy of excitatory synapses (between an hour to several weeks) [67,68]. It is believed to be a mechanism through which memories are formed [69]. In all, dynorphins may act as neurotransmitter and neuromodulator at the synapse MF-CA3 pyramidal cells.

Mossy Fibers Express Neurotrophins and Trophic Activities

In 1952, Rita Levi-Montalcini characterized a soluble factor originating from tumors that induces neuritic growth of sensori neurons in culture. This factor termed "nerve growth factor" (NGF) was later isolated and purified from salivary gland of mouse [70]. NGF was the first member of a class of molecules essential for the development, maintenance and survival of nerve cells, defined as trophic factors. Trophic factors are molecules critical for the development and functioning of the nervous system. They regulate a wide range of biological processes, including neuronal survival, proliferation and migration, axonal and dendritic outgrowth and patterning, synapse strength and plasticity, injury protection, as well as controlling the activity of ion channels and neurotransmitter receptors. Besides their diverse roles in the nervous system, they are also involved in vascular and tumor biology [71]. NGF was the first member of a family of trophic factors originating from a common ancestral gene, the neurotrophins. The neurotrophin family of trophic factors includes brain-derived neurotrophic factor (BDNF), neurotrophin-3 (NT-3) and NT-4/5 [72]. Neurotrophins act through a family of receptors composed of high affinity binding sites, the trk family of tyrosine kinase receptors and a low affinity binding site, p75. Trk-A is NGF's high affinity binding site, trk-B BDNF's high affinity binding site and trk-C NT3's high affinity binding site [73-75]. Other molecules with trophic activities have been isolated and characterized, like the ciliary neurotrophic factor and fibroblast growth factor [76,77].

Neurotrophins are widely distributed in the central nervous system (CNS) and highly expressed in the hippocampus [78-80]. The distribution of NGF, BDNF and NT3 in the hippocampus is highly specific [78]. NGF is mainly express in neurons of the pyramidal layer, *stratum oriens* and hilus of the DG [78,81,82]. The highest levels of messenger for BDNF are found in the pyramidal cell layers of CA2 and CA3, and in the DG [83]. NT-3 mRNAs are confined in the medial area of CA1 and CA2 and in the granule cell layer of the DG, whereas the regions CA3 and hilus do not express NT-3 [78,83-85]. In the hippocampus, gene coding for the trk-B and trk-C are expressed mainly by pyramidal and granule cells [86,87]. The low affinity site p75 is expressed at low level by the neurons of the hippocampus [88]. Trophic factors and activities were reported in MFTs and MFSs supporting the importance of trophic factors in the physiopathology of the MF synapse, particularly BDNF [89,90].

Desmoplakin is Expressed by Granule Cells of the Hippocampus

Desmoplakin is a component of desmosomal tight junctions in peripheral tissues [91]. Desmoplakin mRNA is expressed solely in the DG [92]. Desmoplakin may link intermediate filaments to membrane proteins at MF synapses.

Zinc is Enriched in Granule Cells and Mossy Fibers

Studies in the 1950s reported the presence of high concentrations of zinc in the DG and region of projection of the MFs in the CA3 region, the *stratum lucidum*, after staining of brain sections by dithizone (diphenylthiocarbamate) or Timm's staining [92,93]. Timm's staining is a histological procedure for staining zinc in tissue section, including the brain. During Timm's staining, zinc ions are precipitated as black aggregates of zinc-sulfide, after exposure of the tissue to a solution of sulfide ions [94]. These aggregates of zinc-sulfide are visible in optical microscopy. In 1962, McLardy reported, using a modified Timm's staining protocol, black aggregates of zinc-sulfide at the apical level of the dendritic spines of CA3 pyramidal cells, on transversal sections of guinea pig hippocampus [95]. In 1967, Haug observed sections of rat hippocampus after Timm's staining by electron microscopy. The author reported black aggregates of zinc-sulfide exclusively in the MF ending nerves, as in CA3 region [96]. The presence of high concentration of zinc in MFTs was confirmed by Clairborne et al. (1989) who reported high concentration of zinc in MFS preparations [97].

These data show that the granule cells and MFs are labeled with Timm's staining and therefore are enriched in zinc (figure 3).

However, Timm's staining and other histological procedures staining zinc do not stain the total zinc contained in a given tissue, rather they stain a fraction of this zinc, referred to as "histo-reactive" zinc. Further, dithizone and Timm's staining are not specific of zinc labeling. They label other metals, like heavy and transition metals. The presence of zinc, in the hippocampus and particularly in the granule cells and MFTs, is confirmed by the following experiments. Autoradiographic studies with a radioactive zinc isotope, zinc-65, show a similar staining to the ones obtained from dithizone and Timm's stainings [98]. Preliminary labeling with dithizone or the use of zinc chelating agents prevent the staining of zinc on brain sections by Timm's staining [99,100]. Electrical stimulation and 30 mM potassium depolarization in the MF region, *in vivo*, evoke the release of endogenous zinc in rat [101-104]. Released zinc was assayed by atomic absorption spectroscopy (AAS). Electrical stimulation and 30 mM potassium depolarization in the MF region is followed by a decrease in Timm's staining in the CA3 regions from these animals [94,101]. Assay of zinc by AAS from fractions enriched in MFSs, confirms that the MFTs are enriched in zinc [32]. Further, after hypo-osmotic choc of fractions enriched in MFSs, most of the zinc is recover in the cytosolic fraction [105]. In all, the granule cells and MFTs are enriched in zinc. However, these data do not exclude the colocalization of zinc with other metals in the granule cells and MFTs.

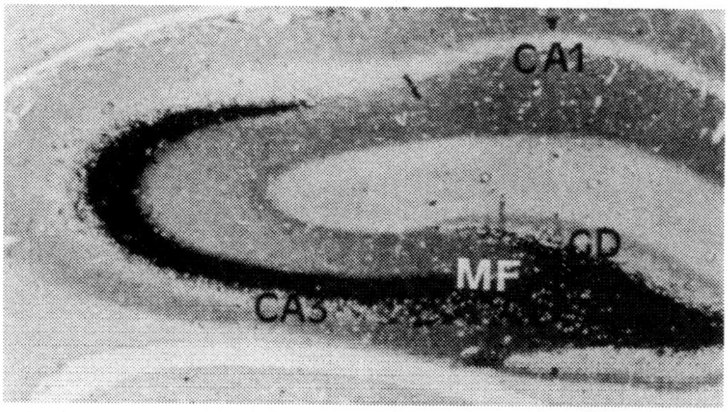

Figure 3. Timm's staining of adult hippocampal sections. Adult rat brains were fixed with paraformaldehyde, processed for histology and Timm's staining. Timm's staining is a histological procedure for staining zinc in tissue section, including the brain. In the hippocampus, the granule cells are the nerve cells of the principal layer of the dentate gyrus (DG), the granule cell layer. Their axons, the mossy fibers (MFs), project to the *Cornu Ammonis* (CA) region CA3 of the hippocampus and establish synaptic contacts with the dendritic spines of pyramidal cells. The granule cells and MF terminals are enriched in zinc. In hippocampal sections from adult rats, Timm's staining labels the DG and the region CA3, revealing the presence of zinc in these regions. These data show that the granule cells and MF terminals are labeled with Timm's staining and therefore are enriched in Zinc.

Determination of zinc concentration by AAS reveals that zinc concentration in the hippocampus is in the range of 240 ppm, 3 times higher than in the other brain regions. This corresponds to approximately 15% of the total zinc in the brain [106]. This conclusion was contradicted by other studies which show that the hippocampus has similar concentration of zinc than other brain regions, ranging from 60-120 ppm (130 μM) [107]. The concentration of zinc seems thus not higher in the hippocampus than in other brain regions. In contrast, studies from microdissected areas of the hippocampus reveal that the concentration of zinc in the region of the MFTs is in the range of 220-300 μM, corresponding to 8% of zinc present in the hippocampus, in rat [108]. Quantitative analysis of zinc by AAS from MFS preparations reported that between 35-50% of the zinc from homogenate of hippocampus is recovered in the P1 pellet, enriched in MFSs [105,107] and that fractions enriched in MFSs are several fold more enriched in zinc than the homogenate and fractions enriched in "small" synaptosomes [30,32,109]. This shows that the region of the MFTs is enriched in zinc. Zinc is considered a marker for granule cells and MFTs.

Zinc is present in almost all the compartments of the cells and organelles where it is associated with metalloproteins and metalloenzymes [110]. In the CNS, Timm (1958) noted the parallel between the distribution of histo-reactive zinc and glutamatergic pathways in the brain [94]. An observation later confirmed in numerous glutamatergic pathways [111-113]. Glu dehydrogenase, the biosynthetic enzyme for Glu, is inhibited by low concentration in zinc (1 nM) [114]. This suggests that zinc is mostly in a bound form in those nerve cells, and particularly in granule cells and MFs. So that it does not inhibit synaptic transmission. In support to this contention, no efflux of zinc-65 is detected from pre-labeled fractions enriched in synaptosomes [115]. Ibata and Otsuka (1969) reported, by electron microscopy, Timm's staining in the synaptic vesicles [116]. Thus, zinc is most likely in a bound form in granule cells and MFs, and histo-reactive zinc is localized within synaptic vesicles and may play a role during nerve activity in granule cells. In granule cells, candidates binding zinc must reach a stoechiometry proportional to the zinc concentration. This to insure that zinc is in a bound form and does not inhibit the synthesis of Glu, necessary for synaptic transmission. The nature of the zinc binding molecules and their distribution in MF synapses remain to be determined.

In granule cells and MFs, Crawford and Connor (1973) proposed that zinc may be bound to Glu [38]. There are also various zinc binding molecules and proteins, candidates for binding zinc in granule cells and MFs; among them, adenosine triphosphate (ATP), metalloproteins, metalloenzymes, like Glu dehydrogenase [117], NGF [118-120], pro-insulin [120], opioid peptides [121] and also GABA [122]. Itch et al. (1983) reported binding of zinc with proteins ranging between 15,000 and 210,000 Daltons [123]. Among these substances, Glu dehydrogenase is not a likely candidate to bind zinc present in MFs, as it is present in low quantities in glutamatergic terminals and particularly in MFTs [124] and it is localized primarily in mitochondria. Trophic factors may represent likely candidates, as trophic activities have been reported to be enriched in MFTs [89].

The presence of high quantities of zinc in granule cells and MFs raises the question of its involvement in the synapse MF-CA3 pyramidal cells. The presence of zinc in MF synaptic vesicles [116], where it is detected in core dense synaptic vesicles, suggests that it is involved in synaptic transmission [98]. In support of this contention, Glu and zinc have been reported to be colocalized in synaptic vesicles [125], zinc has been reported to be released from MFTs in hippocampal slices [101-104,126,127], it is preferentially transported in granule cells and MFTs [115,127] and zinc interacts with different types of glutamatergic and GABAergic receptors [128-131]. These data suggest that zinc may be released by the MF synapses, where it may play a role as neuromediator, acting both pre- and post-synaptically. Zinc may be mediating the activity of Glu and GABA receptors. Particularly, it is an antagonist non-competitive of the N-methyl D-aspartate (NMDA) receptor [132-134].

In all, the region of the MFTs is enriched in zinc and zinc is considered a marker of granule cells and MFTs. In granule cells and MFs, zinc is most likely in a bound form, and histo-reactive zinc is localized within synaptic vesicles. The nature of the zinc binding molecules and their distribution in MF synapses remain to be determined. Zinc may play a role during nerve activity in MFTs.

Conclusion

The granule cells are the nerve cells of the main layer of the hippocampal DG, the granule cell layer or *stratum granulosum*. Their axons, the MFs, project to the pyramidal cells of the CA3 region and establish synaptic contact in a region referred as the *stratum lucidum*. The synapses MF-CA3 pyramidal cells elicit unique histological and biochemical features. They have a large size, up to 10 μm diameter. The MF synapses are enriched in multiple chemical substances, like opioid peptides, trophic factors and zinc. The large size of the MFTs allows their isolation from other cellular structures, including other nerve terminals, by subcellular fractionation. MFS preparations provide a model of choice to study the MFTs *ex vivo*.

The granule cells are glutamatergic excitatory. Opioid peptides and zinc play a role in synaptic transmission at the MF-CA3 synapse. Zinc is most likely in a bound form in granule cells and MFs. The nature of the zinc binding molecules and their distribution in MF synapses remain to be determined. More recently, GABA-immunoreactivity was identified in MFTs [135]. GABA is the main inhibitory neurotransmitter of the nervous system and the neurotransmitter of interneurons [136,137]. The existence of an inhibitory amino acid transmitter in an excitatory glutamatergic nerve cell population raises the question of the role of GABA in MF terminals. Future studies will aim at identifying and characterizing the factors content in the MFTs, and their functions in synaptic transmission and physiopathology of the hippocampus.

Acknowledgments

Chapter 4, figures 2 and 3, are reprinted, with permission, from *J Neurochem*, Vol 62, Taupin P, Zini S, Cesselin F, Ben-Ari Y, Roisin MP, Subcellular fractionation on Percoll gradient of mossy fiber synaptosomes: morphological and biochemical characterization in control and degranulated rat hippocampus, Pages 1586-95, Copyright (1994), Wiley-Blackwell, Inc.

REFERENCES

[1] Amaral DG, Witter MP. (1989) The three-dimensional organization of the hippocampal formation: a review of anatomical data. *Neurosci. 31*, 571-91.

[2] Amaral DG, Insausti R. Hippocampal formation. In: *The human nervous system* (Paxinos G, ed), pp711-755. New York: Academic (1990).

[3] Andersen P, Bliss TV, Lomo T, Olsen LI, Skrede KK. (1969) Lamellar organization of hippocampal excitatory pathways. *Acta Physiol Scand. 76*, 4A-5A.

[4] Gaarskjaer FB. (1986) The organization and development of the hippocampal mossy fiber system. *Brain Res. 396*, 335-57.

[5] Frotscher M. (1985) Mossy fibres form synapses with identified pyramidal basket cells in the CA3 region of the guinea-pig hippocampus: a combined Golgi-electron microscope study. *J Neurocytol. 14*, 245-59.

[6] Acsady L, Kamondi A, Sik A, Freund T, Buzsaki G. (1998) GABAergic cells are the major postsynaptic targets of mossy fibers in the rat hippocampus. *J Neurosci. 18*, 3386-403.

[7] Blackstad TW, Kjaerheim A. (1961) Special axo-dendritic synapses in the hippocampal cortex : electron and light microscopic studies on the layer of the mossy fibers. *J. Comp. Neurol. 117*, 133-59.

[8] Kandel ER, Schwartz JH, Jessell TM. *Principles of Neural Science*. Publisher: McGraw-Hill Medical; 4 edition (January 5, 2000).

[9] Hamlyn LH. (1962) The fine structure of the mossy fiber endings in the hippocampus of the rabbit. *J. Anat. (London). 96*, 112-20.

[10] Niklowitz W. (1966) Elektronenmikroskopische untersuchungen am ammonshorn. *Zeitschrift für Zellforschung. 75*, 485-500.

[11] Amaral DG, Dent JA. (1981) Development of the mossy fibers of the dentate gyrus. I. A light and electron microscopic study of the mossy fibers and their expansion. *J Comp Neurol. 195*, 51-86.

[12] Claiborne BJ, Amaral DG, Cowan WM. (1986) A light and electron microscopic analysis of the mossy fibers of the rat dentate gyrus. *J Comp Neurol. 246*, 435-58.

[13] Braitenberg V, Schüz A. Some anatomical comments on the hippocampus. In *Neurobiology of the hippocampus*. Edited by W. Seifert. Academic Press, 21-37 (1983).

[14] Whittaker VP. (1993) Thirty years of synaptosome research. *J Neurocytol. 22*, 735-42.

[15] De Robertis E, Pellegrino De Iraldi A, Rodriguez De Lorez Arnaiz G, Gomez J. (1961) On the isolation of nerve endings and synaptic vesicles. *J Biophys Biochem Cytol. 9*, 229-35.

[16] Gray EG, Whittaker VP. (1962) The isolation of nerve endings from brain: an electron-microscopic study of cell fragments derived by homogenization and centrifugation. *J Anat (Lond.). 96*, 79-87.

[17] Robert F, Booth G, Clark JB. (1978) A rapid method for the preparation of relatively pure metabolically competent synaptosomes from rat brain. *Biochem J. 176*, 365-70.

[18] Docherty M, Bradford HF, Wu JY. (1987) The preparation of highly purified GABAergic and cholinergic synaptosomes from mammalian brain. *Neurosci Lett. 81*, 232-8.

[19] Dunkley PR, Jarvie PE, Heath JW, Kidd GJ, Rostas JAP. (1986) A rapid method for isolation of synaptosomes on percoll gradients. *Brain Res. 372*, 115-29.

[20] Docherty M, Bradford HF, Cash CD, Ehret M, Maitre M, Joh TH. (1991) Isolation of monoaminergic synaptosomes from rat brain by immunomagnetophoresis. *J Neurochem. 56*, 1569-80.

[21] Wolf ME, Zigmond MJ, Kapatos G. (1989) Tyrosine hydroxylase content of residual striatal dopamine nerve terminals following 6-hydroxydopamine administration: a flow cytometric study. *J Neurochem. 53*, 879-85.

[22] Wolf ME, Kapatos G. (1989) Flow cytometric analysis of rat striatal nerve terminals. *J Neurosci. 9*, 94-105.

[23] Wolf ME, Granneman JG, Kapatos G. (1991) Characterization of the distribution of G alpha o in rat striatal synaptosomes and its colocalization with tyrosine hydroxylase. *Synapse. 9*, 66-74.

[24] Gylys KH, Fein JA, Cole GM. (2000) Quantitative characterization of crude synaptosomal fraction (P-2) components by flow cytometry. *J Neurosci Res. 61*, 186-92.

[25] Gylys KH, Fein JA, Yang F, Cole GM. (2004) Enrichment of presynaptic and postsynaptic markers by size-based gating analysis of synaptosome preparations from rat and human cortex. *Cytometry A. 60*, 90-6.

[26] Smogorzewski M, Ni Z, Massry SG. (1995) Function and metabolism of brain synaptosomes in chronic renal failure. *Artif Organs. 19*, 795-800.

[27] Raiteri L, Raiteri M. (2000) Synaptosomes still viable after 25 years of superfusion. *Neurochem Res. 25*, 1265-74.

[28] Sato Y, Yamanaka H, Toda T, Shinohara Y, Endo T. (2005) Comparison of hippocampal synaptosome proteins in young-adult and aged rats. *Neurosci Lett. 382*, 22-6.

[29] Gylys KH, Fein JA, Yang F, Miller CA, Cole GM. (2007) Increased cholesterol in Abeta-positive nerve terminals from Alzheimer's disease cortex. *Neurobiol Aging. 28*, 8-17.

[30] Terrian DM., Johnston D, Claiborne BJ, Ansah-Yiadom R, Strittmatter WJ, Rea MA. (1988) Glutamate and dynorphin release from a subcellular fraction enriched in hippocampal mossy fiber synaptosomes. *Brain Res Bull. 21*, 343-51.

[31] Terrian DM, Gannon RL, Rea MA. (1990) Glutamate is the endogenous amino acid selectively released by rat hippocampal mossy fiber synaptosomes concomitantly with prodynorphin-derived peptides. *Neurochemical Res. 15*, 1-5.

[32] Taupin P, Zini S, Cesselin F, Ben-Ari Y, Roisin MP. (1994) Subcellular fractionation on Percoll gradient of mossy fiber synaptosomes: morphological and biochemical characterization in control and degranulated rat hippocampus. *J Neurochem. 62*, 1586-95.

[33] Chicurel ME, Terrian DM, Potter H. (1993) mRNA at the synapse: analysis of a synaptosomal preparation enriched in hippocampal dendritic spines. *J Neurosci. 13*, 4054-63.

[34] Kiebler MA, Lopez-Garcia JC, Leopold PL. (1999) Purification and characterization of rat hippocampal CA3-dendritic spines associated with mossy fiber terminals. *FEBS Lett. 445*, 80-6.

[35] Curtis DR, Johnston GA. (1974) Amino acid transmitters in the mammalian central nervous system. *Ergeb Physiol. 69*, 97-188.

[36] Watkins JC. (2000) l-glutamate as a central neurotransmitter: looking back. *Biochem Soc Trans. 28*, 297-309.

[37] Lambert JD, Jones RS, Andreasen M, Jensen MS, Heinemann U. (1989) The role of excitatory amino acids in synaptic transmission in the hippocampus. *Comp Biochem Physiol A. 93*, 195-201.

[38] Crawford I, Connor J. (1973) Localization and release of glutamic acid in relation to the hippocampal mossy fiber pathway. *Nature. 244*, 442-3.

[39] Storm-Mathisen J, Leknes AK, Bore AT, Vaaland JL, Edminson P, Haug FS, Ottersen OP. (1983) First visualization of glutamate and GABA in neurones by immunochemistry. *Nature. 301*, 517-20.

[40] Lanthorn TH, Ganong AH, Cotman CW. (1984) 2-amino-4-phosphonobutyrate selectively blocks mossy fiber-CA3 responses in guinea pig but not rat hippocampus. *Brain Res. 290*, 174-8.

[41] Cotman CW, Flatman JA, Ganong AH, Perkins MN. (1986) Effects of excitatory amino acid antagonists on evoked and spontaneous excitatory potentials in guinea-pig hippocampus. *J. Physiol (London). 378*, 403-15.

[42] Neuman RS, Ben-Ari Y, Gho M, Cherubini E. (1988) Blockade of excitatory synaptic transmission by 6-cyano-7-nitroquinoxaline-2,3-dione (CNQX) in the hippocampus in vitro. *Neurosci Lett. 92*, 64-8.

[43] Foster AC, Mena EE, Monaghan DT, Cotman CW. (1981) Synaptic localization of kainic acid binding sites. *Nature. 289*, 73-5.

[44] Tremblay E, Represa A, Ben-Ari Y. (1985) Autoradiographic localization of kainic acid binding sites in the human hippocampus. *Brain Res. 343*, 378-82.

[45] Represa A, Tremblay E, Schoevart D, Ben-Ari Y. (1986) Development of high affinity kainate binding sites in human and rat hippocampi. *Brain Res. 384*, 170-4.

[46] Cotman CW, Monaghan DT, Ottersen OP, Storm-Mathisen J. (1987) Anatomical organization of excitatory amino acid receptors and their pathways. *TINS. 10*, 273-80.

[47] Dessi F, Represa A, Ben-Ari Y. (1991) Effects of neonatal γ- ray irradiation on rat hippocampus- II. Development of excitatory amino acid binding sites. *Neurosci. 42*, 151-7.

[48] Gannon RL, Terrian DM. (1991) Presynaptic modulation of glutamate and dynorphin release by excitatory amino acids in the guinea-pig hippocampus. *Neurosci. 41*, 401-10.

[49] Masu M, Tanabe Y, Tsuchida K, Shigemoto R, Nakanishi S. (1991) Sequence and expression of a metabotropic glutamate receptor. *Nature. 349*, 760-5.

[50] Hughes J, Smith TW, Kosterlitz HW, Fothergill LA., Morgan BA, Morris HR. (1975) Identification of two related pentapeptides from the brain with potent opiate agonist activity. *Nature. 258*, 577-9.

[51] Smith AP, Lee NM. (1988) Pharmacology of dynorphin. *Ann rev Pharmacol Toxicol. 28*, 123-40.

[52] Hollt V. (1986) Opioid peptide processing and receptor selectivity. *Ann Rev Pharmacol Toxicol. 26*, 59-77.

[53] Docherty K, Steiner DF. (1982) Post-translational proteolysis in polypeptide hormone biosynthesis. *Ann Rev Physiol., 44*, 625-38.

[54] Sar M, Stumpf WE, Miller RJ, Chang KJ, Cuatrecasas P. (1978) Immunohistochemical localization of enkephalin in rat brain and spinal cord. *J Comp Neurol. 182*, 17-38.

[55] Weber E, Evans C, Barchas JD. (1982) Predominance of the amino-terminal octapeptide fragment of dynorphin in rat brain regions. *Nature. 299*, 77-9.

[56] Simatov R, Snowman AM, Snyder SH. (1976) A morphine-like factor enkephalin' in rat brain: subcellular localization. *Brain Res. 107*, 650-7.

[57] Weber E, Roth KA, Barchas JD. (1982) Immunohistochemical distribution of α-neo-endorphin/dynorphin neuronal systems in rat brain: Evidence for colocalization. *Proc Natl Sci U S A. 79*, 3062-6.

[58] Chavkin C, Bakhit C, Weber E, Bloom FE. (1983) Relative contents and concomitant release of prodynorphin/neoendorphin-derived peptides in rat hippocampus. *Proc Natl Acad Sci U S A. 80*, 7669-73.

[59] McGinty JF, Henriksen SJ, Goldstein A, Terenius L, Bloom FE. (1983) Dynorphin is contained within hippocampal mossy fibers: immunochemical alterations after kainic acid administration and colchicine induced neurotoxicity. *Proc Natl Acad Sci USA. 80*, 589-93.

[60] Hoffman DW, Zamir N. (1984) Localization and quantitation of dynorphin B in the rat hippocampus. *Brain Res. 324*, 354-7.

[61] Van Daal JHHM., Valentijn JA, Jenks BG, Van Abeelen JHF. (1991) Dynorphin B in the mouse hippocampus: an ultrastructural survey. *Neurosci Res Comm. 8*, 37-40.

[62] Wagner JJ, Evans CJ, Chavkin C. (1991) Focal stimulation of the mossy fibers releases endogenous dynorphins that bind k1-opioid receptors in guinea pig hippocampus. *J Neurochem. 57*, 333-43.

[63] Conner-Kerr TA, Simmons DR, Peterson GM, Terrian DM. (1993) Evidence for the corelease of dynorphin and glutamate from rat hippocampal mossy fiber terminals. *J Neurochem. 61*, 627-36.

[64] McLean S, Rothman RB., Jacobson AE., Rice KC, Herkenham M. (1987) Distribution of opiate receptor subtypes and enkephalin and dynorphin immunoreactivity in the hippocampus of squirrel, guinea pig, rat and hamster. *J Comp Neurol. 255*, 497-510.

[65] Weisskopf MG., Zalutsky RA, Nicoll RA. (1993) The opioid peptide dynorphin mediates heterosynaptic depression of hippocampal mossy fibre synapses and modulates long-term potentiation. *Nature. 362*, 423-7.

[66] Cohen GA, Doze VA, Madison DV. (1992) Opioid inhibition of GABA release from presynaptic terminals of rat hippocampal interneurons. *Neuron. 9*, 325-35.

[67] Bliss TV, Lomo T. (1973) Long-lasting potentiation of synaptic transmission in the dentate area of the anaesthetized rabbit following stimulation of the perforant path. *J Physiol. 232*, 331-56.

[68] Lomo T. (2003) The discovery of long-term potentiation. *Philos Trans R Soc Lond B Biol Sci. 358*, 617-20.

[69] Malenka RC, Nicoll RA. (1999) Long-term potentiation--a decade of progress? *Science. 285*, 1870-4.

[70] Levi-Montalcini R. (1987) The nerve growth factor: thirty-five years later. *EMBO J. 6*, 1145-54.

[71] Huang EJ, Reichardt LF. (2001) Neurotrophins: roles in neuronal development and function. *Annu Rev Neurosci. 24*, 677-736.

[72] Reichardt LF. (2006) Neurotrophin-regulated signalling pathways. *Philos Trans R Soc Lond B Biol Sci. 361*, 1545-64.

[73] Patapoutian A, Reichardt LF. (2001) Trk receptors, mediators of neurotrophin action. *Curr Opin Neurobiol. 11*, 272-80.

[74] Huang EJ, Reichardt LF. (2003) Trk receptors: roles in neuronal signal transduction. *Annu Rev Biochem. 72*, 609-42.

[75] Hennigan A, O'callaghan RM, Kelly AM. (2007) Neurotrophins and their receptors: roles in plasticity, neurodegeneration and neuroprotection. *Biochem Soc Trans. 35*, 424-7.

[76] Barbin G, Manthorpe M, Varon S. (1984) Purification of the chick eye ciliary neuronotrophic factor. *J Neurochem. 43*, 1468-78.

[77] Bohlen P, Baird A, Esch F, Ling N, Gospodarowicz D. (1984) Isolation and partial molecular characterization of pituitary fibroblast growth factor. *Proc Natl Acad Sci U S A. 81*, 5364-8.

[78] Ernfors P, Ibanez CF, Ebendal T, Olson L, Persson H. (1990) Molecular cloning and neurotrophic activities of a protein with structural similarities to nerve growth factor: developmental and topographical expression in the brain. *Proc Natl Acad Sci U S A. 87*, 5454-8.

[79] Hohn A, Leibrock J, Bailey K, Barde YA. (1990) Identification and characterization of a novel member of the nerve growth factor/brain-derived neurotrophic factor family. *Nature. 344*, 339-41.

[80] Maisonpierre PC, Belluscio L, Squinto S, Ip NY, Furth ME, Lindsay RM, Yancopoulos GD. (1990) Neurotrophin-3 : a neurotrophic factor related to NGF and BDNF. *Science. 247*, 1446-51.

[81] Ayer-LeLievre C, Olson L, Seiger A, Ebendal T, Seiger A, Person H. (1988) Expression of the ß-nerve growth factor in hippocampal neurons. *Science. 240*, 1339-41.

[82] Gall CM, Isackson PJ. (1989) Limbic seizures increase neuronal production of messenger RNA for nerve growth factor. *Science. 245*, 758-60.

[83] Phillips HS, Hains JM, Laramee GR, Rosenthal A, Winslow JW. (1990) Widespread expression of BDNF but not NT-3 by target areas of basal forebrain cholinergic neurons. *Science. 250*, 290-4.

[84] Friedman WJ, Ernfors P, Persson H. (1991) Transient and persistent expression of NT-3/HDNF mRNA in the rat brain during postnatal development. *J Neurosci. 11*, 1577-84.

[85] Vigers AJ, Baquet ZC, Jones KR. (2000) Expression of neurotrophin-3 in the mouse forebrain: insights from a targeted LacZ reporter. *J Comp Neurol. 416*, 398-415.

[86] Klein R, Conway D, Parada LF, Barbacid M. (1990) The trk B tyrosine protein kinase gene codes for a second neurogenic receptor that lacks the catalytic domain. *Cell. 61*, 647-56.

[87] Lamballe F, Klein R, Barbacid M. (1991) trkC, a new member of tyrosine protein kinases, is a receptor for neurotrophin-3. *Cell. 66*, 967-79.

[88] Buck CR., Martinez HJ, Black IB, Chao MV. (1987) Developmentally regulated expression of the nerve growth factor receptor gene in the periphery and brain. *Proc Natl Acad Sci U S A. 84*, 3060-3.

[89] Taupin P, Roisin MP, Ben-Ari Y, Barbin G. (1994) A fraction enriched in rat hippocampal mossy fibre synaptosomes contains trophic activities. *Neuroreport. 5*, 1353-5.

[90] Danzer SC, McNamara JO. (2004) Localization of brain-derived neurotrophic factor to distinct terminals of mossy fiber axons implies regulation of both excitation and feedforward inhibition of CA3 pyramidal cells. *J Neurosci. 24*, 11346-55.

[91] Kowalczyk AP, Borgwardt JE, Green KJ. (1996) Analysis of desmosomal cadherin-adhesive function and stoichiometry of desmosomal cadherin-plakoglobin complexes. *J Invest Dermatol. 107*, 293-300.

[92] Lein ES, Zhao X, Gage FH. (2004) Defining a molecular atlas of the hippocampus using DNA microarrays and high-throughput in situ hybridization. *J Neurosci. 24*, 3879-89.

[93] Maske H. (1955) Uber den topographischen nachweis von zink im ammonshorn verschiedener saugetiere. *Naturwissenschaften. 42*, 424.

[94] Timm F. (1958) Zur histochemie des ammon-shornsgebietes. *Z Zellforsch. 48*, 548-55.

[95] McLardy T. (1962) Zinc enzymes and the hippocampal mossy fibre system. *Nature. 194*, 300-2.

[96] Haug FMS. (1967) Electron microscopical localization of the zinc in hippocampal mossy fiber synapses by a modified sulfide silver procedure. *Histochimie. 8*, 355-68.

[97] Claiborne BJ, Rea MA, Terrian DM. (1989) Detection of zinc in isolated nerve terminals using a modified Timm's sulfide-silver method. *J Neurosci Methods. 30*, 17-22.

[98] Von Euler C. On the significance of the high zinc content in the hippocampal formation. In: *Physiologie de L'Hippocampe. P. Passouant,] ed. Editions du Centre National de la Recherche Scientifique* (Coll. Intern. du C.N.R.S. No. 107), Paris, 135-145 (1962).

[99] Danscher G, Haug FMS, Fredens K. (1973) Effect of diethyldithiocarbamate (DEDTC) on sulphide silver stained boutons, reversible blocking of Timm's sulphide silver stain for "heavy" metals in DEDTC treated rats (light microscopy). *Exp Brain Res. 16*, 521-32.

[100] Fjerdingstad E, Danscher G, Fjerdingstad EJ. (1977) Changes in zinc and lead content of rat hippocampus and whole brain following intravital dithizone treatment as determined by flameless atomic absorption spectrophotometry. *Brain Res. 130*, 369-73.

[101] Sloviter RS. (1982) A simplified Timm stain procedure compatible with formaldehyde fixation and routine paraffin embedding of rat brain. *Brain Res Bull. 8*, 771-4.

[102] Slovitter RS. (1984) A selective loss of Timm staining in the hippocampal mossy fiber pathway accompanies electrically induced hippocampal granule cell seizure activity in rats. In: Frederickson C.J. (ed) *Neurobiology of zinc*. AR Liss, New York (1984).

[103] Charton G, Rovira C, Ben-Ari Y, Leviel V. (1985) Spontaneous and evoked release of endogenous Zn2+ in the hippocampal mossy fiber zone of the rat in situ. *Exp Brain Res. 58*, 202-5.

[104] Aniksztejn L, Charton G, Ben-Ari Y. (1987) Selective release of endogenous zinc from the hippocampal mossy fibers in situ. *Brain Res. 404*, 58-64.

[105] Sato SM, Frazier JM, Goldberg AM. (1984) The distribution and binding of zinc in the hippocampus. *J Neurosci. 4*, 1662-70.

[106] Fjerdingstad E, Danscher G, Fjerdingstad EJ. (1974) Zinc content in hippocampus and whole brain of normal rats. *Brain Res, 79*, 338-42.

[107] Crawford Il, Connor JD. (1972) Zinc in maturing rat brain : hippocampal concentration and localization. *J. Neurochem. 19*, 1451-8.

[108] Frederickson CJ, Klitenick MA, Manton WI, Kirkpatrick JB. (1983) Cytoarchitectonic distribution of zinc in the hippocampus of man and rat. *Brain Res. 273*, 335-9.

[109] Crawford IL, Harris NF. Distribution and accumulation of zinc in whole brain and subcellular fractions of hippocampal homogenates. *The Neurobiology of Zinc.*, Part A: Physiochemistry, Anatomy, and Techniques.157-171 (1984).

[110] Vallee BL, Falchuk KH. (1993) The biochemical basis of zinc physiology. *Physiol. Rev. 73*, 79-118.

[111] Friedman B, Price JL. (1984) Fiber systems in the olfactory bulb and cortex : a study in adult and developing rats, using the Timm method with the light and electron microscope. *J Comp Neurol. 223*, 88-109.

[112] Perez-Clausell J, Danscher G. (1985) Intravesicular localization of zinc in rat telencephalic boutons. A histochemical study. *Brain Res. 337*, 91-8.

[113] Slomianka L. (1992) Neurons of origin of zinc-containing pathways and the distribution of zinc-containing boutons in the hippocampal region of the rat. *Neurosci. 48*, 325-52.

[114] Bell ET, Stilwell AM, Bell JE. (1987) Interaction of Zn2+ and Eu3+ with bovine liver glutamate dehydrogenase. *Biochem J. 246*, 199-203.

[115] Wensink J, Molenaar AJ, Woroniecka UD, Van den Hamer CJA. (1988) Zinc uptake into synaptosomes. *J Neurochem. 50*, 782-9.

[116] Ibata Y, Otsuka N. (1969) Electron microscopic demonstration of zinc in the hippocampal formation using sulfide-silver technique. *J Histochem Cytochem. 17*, 171-5.

[117] Chen R, Ganther HE. (1975) Relative cadnium-binding capacity of metallothionein and other cytosolic fractions in various tissues of the rat. Environ. *Physiol Biochem. 5*, 378-88.

[118] Stewart GR, Frederickson CJ, Howell GA, Gage FH. (1984) Cholinergic denervation-induced increase of chelatable zinc in mossy-fiber region of the hippocampal formation. *Brain Res. 290*, 43-51.

[119] Greene LA, Shooter EM. (1980) The nerve growth factor: biochemistry, synthesis and mechanism. *Ann Rev Neurosci. 3*, 353-402.

[120] Pattison SE, Dunn F. (1975) On the relationship of zinc ion to the structure and function of the 7S nerve growth factor protein. *Biochemistry. 14*, 2733-8.

[121] Steengaard-Pedersen K, Larsson LI. (1981) Inhibition of opiate receptor binding by zinc ions: possible physiological importance in the hippocampus. *Peptides. 2 (suppl. 1)*, 27-35.

[122] Xie X, Smart TG. (1991) A physiological role for endogenous zinc in rat hippocampal synaptic neurotransmission. *Nature. 349*, 521-4.

[123] Itoh M, Ebadi M, Swanson S. (1983) The presence of zinc-binding proteins in brain. *J Neurochem. 41*, 823-9.

[124] Vallee BL. Metal and enzyme interactions: correlation of composition, function, and structure. In: Boyer, F.G., Lardy, N and Myrback, K. (eds) *The Enzymes*. Academic Press, New York-London, 3, 225-276 (1960).

[125] Martinez-Guijarro FJ, Soriano E, Del Rio JA, Lopez-Garcia C. (1991) Zinc-positive boutons in the cerebral cortex of lizards show glutamate immunoreactivity. *J Neurocytol. 20*, 834-43.

[126] Assaf SY, Chung SH. (1984) Release of endogenous Zn2+ from brain tissue during activity. *Nature. 308*, 734-6.

[127] Howell GA, Welch MG, Frederickson CJ. (1984) Stimulation-induced uptake and release of zinc in hippocampal slices. *Nature. 308*, 736-8.

[128] Westbrook GL, Mayer ML. (1987) Micromolar concentrations of Zn2+ antagonize NMDA and GABA responses of hippocampal neurons. *Nature. 328*, 640-3.

[129] Mayer ML, Vyklicky L, Westbrook GL. (1989) Modulation of excitatory amino acid receptors by group IIB metal cations in cultured mouse hippocampal neurons. *J Physiol. 415*, 329-50.

[130] Legendre P, Westbrook GL. (1990) The inhibition of single N-methyl-D-aspartate-activated channels by zinc ions on cultured rat neurons. *J Physiol. 429*, 429-49.

[131] Ruiz A, Walker MC, Fabian-Fine R, Kullmann DM. (2004) Endogenous zinc inhibits GABA(A) receptors in a hippocampal pathway. *J Neurophysiol. 91*, 1091-6.

[132] Peters S, Koh J, Choi DW. (1987) Zinc selectively blocks the action of N-methyl-D-aspartate on cortical neurons. *Science. 236*, 589-93.

[133] Koh JY, Choi DW. (1988) Zinc alters excitatory amino acid neurotoxicity on cortical neurons. *J Neurosci. 8*, 2164-71.

[134] Molnar P, Nadler JV. (2001) Synaptically-released zinc inhibits N-methyl-D-aspartate receptor activation at recurrent mossy fiber synapses. *Brain Res. 910*, 205-7.

[135] Sandler R, Smith AD. (1991) Coexistence of GABA and glutamate in mossy fiber terminals of the primate hippocampus: an ultrastructural study. *J Comp Neurol. 303*, 177-92.

[136] Ribak CE, Seress L. (1983) Five types of basket cell in the hippocampal dentate gyrus: a combined Golgi and electron microscopic study. *J Neurocytol. 12*, 577-97.

[137] Seress L, Ribak CE. (1983) GABAergic cells in the dentate gyrus appear to be local circuit and projection neurons. *Exp Brain Res. 50*, 173-82.

Chapter V

The Dale's Principle

Abstract

Neurotransmitters are molecules, synthesized and stored in neurons, that are released during nerve activity, interact with specific receptors in the postsynaptic membrane and relay the transmission of nerve activity. The identification of chemical transmission has the main mode of transmission of nerve activity and acetyl choline as the first neurotransmitter has led to the principle of chemical identity of nerve cells, known as Dale's principle. According to the Dale's principle, an individual neuron releases only one neurotransmitter. Over the years, various neurotransmitters and their mechanisms of action have been identified and characterized in the nervous system. Evidence that multiple neurotransmitters co-exist within the same nerve terminals led to the re-evaluation of the Dale's principle. The existence of multiple neurotransmitters within the same nerve cells has profound consequences for brain functioning and physiopathology of the nervous system.

Introduction

In the nervous system, chemical transmission is the main mode of transmission of nerve activity between nerve cells or nerves cells and other cells, like muscle cells and gland cells [1]. Chemical transmission is mediated by the release of neurotransmitters at the synapses, and their interaction with postsynaptic receptors. In the 1920s and 30s, Otto Loewi and Henri Dale identified chemical transmission as the main mode of transmission of nerve activity and acetyl choline, as the first neurotransmitter [2,3]. Based on this work, Dale proposed the concept of chemical identity of nerve cells that nerve cells are characterized by their neurotransmitter. Dale proposed that nerve cells be classified according to the neurotransmitter they released, e.g., nerve cells using acetyl choline as a neurotransmitter are cholinergic, those using glutamate (glutamic acid, Glu) are glutamatergic and those using y-aminobutyric acid (GABA) are GABAergic [4]. This nomenclature is still in use nowadays.

The principle, known as the Dale's principle, was enounced by John Eccles in reference to Dale's work [5]. It states that "the same chemical transmitter is released from all the synaptic terminals of a neuron" [6]. Eccles further stated that "the same mechanical manufacturing goes on throughout the whole extent of a cell, and that a cell cannot make one kind of transmitter substance for some of its terminals and another kind for others" [7]. According to the Dale's principle, nerve cells release one neurotransmitter. Progress in physiology and the identification of multiple substances characterized as neurotransmitters, within the same nerve terminals, lead researchers to propose that nerve cells may release more than one neurotransmitter [8]. In light of these data, Eccles re-examined the Dale's principle and proposed that "Dale's principle be defined as stating that at all the axonal branches of a neuron, there was liberation of the same transmitter substance or substances" [9]. The Dale's principle supports the chemical identity of nerve cells, rather than whether or not it releases a single neurotransmitter.

Neurotransmitters and Neuromediators

Neurotransmitters are molecules synthesized and stored in neurons that are released during nerve activity, interact with specific receptors in the postsynaptic membrane and relay the transmission of nerve activity [8]. Neuromediators or neuromodulators are substances contained within synapses that are stored in synaptic vesicles. Upon their release, neuromediators act through pre- and/or postsynaptic receptors to modulate the activity of neurotransmitters.

Over the years, various substances have been identified and characterized as neurotransmitters and neuromediators in the nervous system. There are three main types of substances that are neurotransmitters and/or neuromediators in the nervous system: amino acids, monoamines and peptides.

Multiple Neurotransmitters within the Same Nerve Cells

Over the years, there have been numerous studies reporting the co-localization and co-release of substances characterized as neurotransmitters, from the same nerve terminals.

Upon depolarization, GABAergic synaptosomes isolated from the cerebral cortex release Glu and aspartate (aspartic acid, Asp), in addition to GABA [10]. Combinations of two or more neuroactive amino acids, like Glu, Asp, GABA and glycine (Gly), are observed within the same nerve terminals of the vestibular nuclear complex in cat, particularly the following combinations are observed: GABA and Gly, Gly, Asp and Glu, Gly and Asp, and Glu and Asp. This raises the possibility of co-release of two or more amino acids from these synapses [11]. Fast ionotropic amino acid neurotransmitters can also be co-released with neuropeptides [12] and monoamines [13,14].

In the hippocampus, dentate granule cells are excitatory glutamatergic. [15]. In 1991, Sandler and Smith reported the presence of GABA in the ending nerves of granule cells, the mossy fiber terminals (MFTs). The co-localization of Glu and GABA within MFTs was reported from monkey and human tissues, by immunohistochemistry and electron microscopy [16]. GABA is an inhibitory neurotransmitter and the main neurotransmitter of interneurons [17,18]. The existence of GABA in the ending nerves of a population of excitatory glutamatergic nerve cells raises the possibility that GABA may be co-released with Glu and act as a neurotransmitter at the synapse of the MF-pyramidal cells of *Cornu Ammonis* (CA) region CA3. In support to this contention, Glu and GABA are co-released, upon depolarization evoked by high concentration of potassium (50 mM), from fractions enriched in rat mossy fiber synaptosomes (MFSs) [19]. The evoked release of Glu and GABA from MFSs is calcium-dependent, revealing that Glu and GABA could act as co-neurotransmitters at the synapse MF-CA3 pyramidal cells.

GABA and Gly are co-localized and co-released from the same nerve terminals of spinal cord interneurons. Further, in these nerve terminals, the transmitters are present within the same synaptic vesicles and their release activates functionally distinct receptors of their postsynaptic target cells [20]. Glu and GABA also coexist in a small population of neurons of the rat accessory olfactory bulb [21].

This shows that multiple substances characterized as neurotransmitters are co-localized and co-released from the same nerve terminals, and can act as neurotransmitters at the same synapse.

The medium spiny neurons that project from the neostriatum to the globus pallidus and the substantia nigra, *pars reticularis*, are inhibitory GABAergic neurons of the striatum [22-24]. In rat and monkey, these neurons express the high-affinity uptake transporter for Glu and Asp [25,26]. This shows that these neurons possess the high-affinity uptake system for excitatory amino acids without these substances acting as neurotransmitters at this synapse. GABA is synthesized in the cytoplasm of neurons from Glu by Glu decarboxylase (GAD) [27]. The presence high-affinity Glu uptake system on GABAergic neurons could satisfy metabolic demands of striatal medium spiny nerve cells, by providing alternative source of Glu for GABA synthesis. It may also serve as a neuroprotective mechanism against local glutamate toxicity [28]. Alternatively, since high-affinity Glu uptake transporter is considered a marker for glutamatergic neurons, some striato-pallidal and striato-nigral projection neurons may utilize Glu as neurotransmitter [29]. This raises the possibility that Glu and GABA may serve as co-neurotransmitters within the same striatal projection neurons.

This shows that nerve cells possess the machinery to use of multiple substances as neurotransmitters. This further supports the fact that individual nerve cells may have multiple neurotransmitters.

Significance of the Co-Release of Multiple Transmitters from the same Nerve Cell Population

The mechanism, function and physiological significance of the co-release of multiple neurotransmitters by the same nerve cells remain to be determined. The co-release of multiple transmitters from the same synapse could support different functions. Among them, the co-release of neurotransmitters from the same presynaptic nerve terminals could i) regulate the membrane conductance changes at the postsynaptic membrane and therefore transmission of nerve activity, ii) regulate metabolic activities of the postsynaptic cells, when one neurotransmitter may act on both ionotropic and metabotropic receptors, iii) enable a feedback control of the transmission; particularly when one neurotransmitter has both pre- and postsynaptic receptors, like GABA [30], and iv) play a neuroprotective function during pathological events, as the expression of one neurotransmitter may be stimulated in an attempt to compensate for neuronal hyperactivity and toxicity.

In support of the latter contention, GAD activity is increased in granule cells and MFs, after kainic acid treatment that triggers experimental seizures [31,32]. As GABA and GABA-mediated inhibition are known to have anticonvulsant activity, an increase in GABA synthesis and release from MFTs during epileptic seizures may represent an attempt by the nervous system to reduce the Glu toxicity on pyramidal cells and return to a normal state [33].

The co-release of multiple transmitters at the same synapse could also provide a redundant mechanism of transmission, made in place during evolution [34]. It could compensate for eventual mutation in one of the transmitters' pathways; particularly when identical types of neurotransmitters are co-released at the same synapses, like Glu and Asp or GABA and Gly.

Alternatively, co-localization of substances known as neurotransmitters may not signify that they all act as neurotransmitter, but may purely play a metabolic, a neuroprotective function or act as neuromodulator [34,35]. Particularly, Glu localized in GABAergic terminals has been shown to modulate GABAergic potentials [36].

On the mechanism level, the control of neural activity at these synapses remains to be understood and involves complex regulatory processes. Particularly, the existence of multiple transmitters within the same neuronal cell population raises the question of whether all synapses from the same nerve cell population contain the same distribution of neurotransmitters and whether different neurotransmitters can be differentially released at different terminals [37]. The significance of the existence of multiple neurotransmitters at the same synapse needs to be evaluated on a case by case basis.

CONCLUSION

The chemical identity of nerve cells proposed by Dale and enounced as a principle by Eccles has been challenged by the discovery of multiple neurotransmitters at the same nerve terminals. The existence of multiple neurotransmitters within individual nerve cells further challenges our understanding of brain functioning, at the network and individual cell levels. For example, in the nervous system, excitatory and inhibitory transmissions are believed to be carried out by separate populations of nerve cells [38]. The presence of an excitatory neurotransmitter, Glu, and inhibitory neurotransmitter, GABA, within the MF synapse not only reveals the existence of "dual" excitatory and inhibitory synapses, but suggests that the functioning of neural networks involves more complex regulatory processes. At the individual cell level, the existence of multiple transmitters within the same neuronal cell population raises the question of whether all the synapses contain the same distribution of neurotransmitters.

It also raises the questions of the mechanisms underlying the synthesis and release of multiple neurotransmitters by individual nerve cells, and the physio- and pathological functions of the co-release of multiple neurotransmitters. The elucidation of these questions may not only have significant consequences for our understanding of the brain functioning and physiopathology, but also for the design of new drugs for the treatment of neurological diseases and disorders.

REFERENCES

[1] Kandel ER, Schwartz JH, Jessell TM. *Principles of Neural Science.* Publisher: McGraw-Hill Medical; 4 edition (January 5, 2000).

[2] Loewi O. (1921) Uber humorale Ubertragbarkeit des Herznervenwirkung. *Pflugers Arch. 189*, 239-42.

[3] Dale HH, Gaddum JH. (1930) Reactions to denervated voluntary muscle and their bearing on the mode of action of parasympathetic and related nerves. *J Physiol (Lond). 70*, 109-44.

[4] Dale HH. (1935) Pharmacology and nerve-endings. *Proc R Soc Med. 28*, 319-32.

[5] Eccles JC. (1986) Chemical transmission and Dale's principle. *Prog Brain Res. 68*, 3-13.

[6] Eccles JC, Fatt P, Koketsu K. (1954) Cholinergic and inhibitory synapses in a pathway from motor-axon collaterals to motoneurones. *J Physiol (Lond). 126*, 524-62.

[7] Eccles JC. (1957) The clinical significance of research work on the chemical transmitter substances of the nervous system. *Med J Aust. 1*, 747-53.

[8] Burnstock G. (1976) Do some nerve cells release more than one transmitter? *Neurosci. 1*, 239-48.

[9] Eccles JC. (1976) From electrical to chemical transmission in the central nervous system. *R. Soc. London Notes and records. 30*, 219-30.

[10] Docherty M, Bradford HF, Wu JY. (1987) Co-release of glutamate and aspartate from cholinergic and GABAergic synaptosomes. *Nature. 330*, 64-6.

[11] Walberg F, Ottersen OP, Rinvik E. (1990) GABA, glycine, aspartate, glutamate and taurine in the vestibular nuclei: an immunocytochemical investigation in the cat. *Exp Brain Res. 79*, 547-63.

[12] Hokfelt T. (1991) Neuropeptides in perspective: the last ten years. *Neuron. 7*, 867-79.

[13] Campbell KJ, Takada M, Hattori T. (1991) Co-localization of tyrosine hydroxylase and glutamate decarboxylase in a subpopulation of single nigrotectal projection neurons. *Brain Res. 558*, 239-44.

[14] Trudeau LE. (2004) Glutamate co-transmission as an emerging concept in monoamine neuron function. *J Psychiatry Neurosci. 29*, 296-310.

[15] Langdon RB, Johnson JW, Barrionuevo G. (1993) Asynchrony of mossy fibre inputs and excitatory postsynaptic currents in rat hippocampus. *J Physiol. 472*, 157-76.

[16] Sandler R, Smith AD. (1991) Coexistence of GABA and glutamate in mossy fiber terminals of the primate hippocampus: an ultrastructural study. *J Comp Neurol. 303*, 177-92.

[17] Ribak CE, Seress L. (1983) Five types of basket cell in the hippocampal dentate gyrus: a combined Golgi and electron microscopic study. *J Neurocytol. 12*, 577-97.

[18] Seress L, Ribak CE. (1983) GABAergic cells in the dentate gyrus appear to be local circuit and projection neurons. *Exp Brain Res. 50*, 173-82.

[19] Taupin P, Ben-Ari Y, Roisin MP. (1994) Subcellular fractionation on Percoll gradient of mossy fiber synaptosomes: evoked release of glutamate, GABA, aspartate and glutamate decarboxylase activity in control and degranulated rat hippocampus. *Brain Res. 644*, 313-21.

[20] Jonas P, Bischofberger J, Sandkuhler J. (1998) Corelease of two fast neurotransmitters at a central synapse. *Science. 281*, 419-24.

[21] Quaglino E, Giustetto M, Panzanelli P, Cantino D, Fasolo A, Sassoe-Pognetto M. (1999) Immunocytochemical localization of glutamate and gamma-aminobutyric acid in the accessory olfactory bulb of the rat. *J Comp Neurol. 408*, 61-72.

[22] Somogyi P, Smith AD. (1979) Projection of neostriatal spiny neurons to the substantia nigra. Application of a combined Golgi-staining and horseradish peroxidase transport procedure at both light and electron microscopic levels. *Brain Res. 178*, 3-15.

[23] Preston RJ, Bishop GA, Kitai ST. (1980) Medium spiny neuron projection from the rat striatum: an intracellular horseradish peroxidase study. *Brain Res. 183*, 253-63.

[24] Kita H, Kitai ST. (1991) Intracellular study of rat globus pallidus neurons: membrane properties and responses to neostriatal, subthalamic and nigral stimulation. *Brain Res. 564*, 296-305.

[25] Kisvarday ZF, Cowey A, Smith AD, Somogyi P. (1989) Interlaminar and lateral excitatory amino acid connections in the striate cortex of monkey. *J Neurosci. 9*, 667-82.

[26] White LE, Hodges HD, Carnes KM, Price JL, Dubinsky JM. (1994) Colocalization of excitatory and inhibitory neurotransmitter markers in striatal projection neurons in the rat. *J Comp Neurol. 339*, 328-40.

[27] Kaufman DL, Houser CR, Tobin AJ. (1991) Two forms of the gamma-aminobutyric acid synthetic enzyme glutamate decarboxylase have distinct intraneuronal distributions and cofactor interactions. *J Neurochem. 56*, 720-3.

[28] Uhl GR. (1992) Neurotransmitter transporters (plus): a promising new gene family. *Trends Neurosci. 15*, 265-8.

[29] Heja L, Karacs K, Kardos J. (2006) Role for GABA and Glu plasma membrane transporters in the interplay of inhibitory and excitatory neurotransmission. *Curr Top Med Chem. 6*, 989-95.

[30] Mohler H. (2006) GABA(A) receptor diversity and pharmacology. *Cell Tissue Res. 326*, 505-16.

[31] Schwarzer C, Sperk G. (1995) Hippocampal granule cells express glutamic acid decarboxylase-67 after limbic seizures in the rat. *Neurosci. 69*, 705-9.

[32] Sloviter RS, Dichter MA, Rachinsky TL, Dean E, Goodman JH, Sollas AL, Martin DL. (1996) Basal expression and induction of glutamate decarboxylase and GABA in excitatory granule cells of the rat and monkey hippocampal dentate gyrus. *J Comp Neurol. 373*, 593-618.

[33] Meldrum BS, Rogawski MA. (2007) Molecular targets for antiepileptic drug development. *Neurotherapeutics. 4*, 18-61.

[34] Somogyi J. (2006) Functional significance of co-localization of GABA and Glu in nerve terminals: a hypothesis. *Curr Top Med Chem. 6*, 969-73.

[35] Seal RP, Edwards RH. (2006) Functional implications of neurotransmitter co-release: glutamate and GABA share the load. *Curr Opin Pharmacol. 6*, 114-9.

[36] Stelzer A, Wong RK. (1989) GABAA responses in hippocampal neurons are potentiated by glutamate. *Nature. 337*, 170-3.

[37] Kandel ER, Gardner D. (1972) The synaptic actions mediated by the different branches of a single neuron. *Res Publ Assoc Res Nerv Ment Dis. 50*, 91-146.

[38] Roberts E. (1991) Living systems are tonically inhibited, autonomous optimizers, and disinhibition coupled to variability generation is their major organizing principle: inhibitory command-control at levels of membrane, genome, metabolism, brain, and society. *Neurochem Res. 16*, 409-21.

Chapter VI

PLASTICITY OF THE GABA PHENOTYPE IN THE NERVOUS SYSTEM

ABSTRACT

Two kinds of fast-acting neurotransmitters exist in the nervous system, excitatory and inhibitory. Excitatory neurotransmitters depolarize the membrane potential of nerve cells and increase their excitability, leading to the propagation of nerve activity. Inhibitory neurotransmitters hyperpolarize the membrane potential and decrease the excitability of target cells. In the vertebrate nervous system, glutamate (glutamic acid, Glu) is the main excitatory neurotransmitter and γ-aminobutyric acid (GABA) the main inhibitory neurotransmitter. In the mature nervous system, GABA is the main neurotransmitter of interneurons. Evidences reveal that, in certain situations, GABA depolarizes the membrane potential of nerve cells, acting as an excitatory neurotransmitter. Glutamatergic neurons may also elicit a GABA phenotype, suggesting that excitatory nerve cells may also contain and use inhibitory neurotransmitters. Hence, nerve cells elicit some forms of plasticity in the expression of their phenotype, particularly the GABA phenotype. This phenotypic plasticity has tremendous implications for our understanding of the development and physiopathology of the nervous system.

INTRODUCTION

GABA is the main inhibitory neurotransmitter of the nervous system. It is the main fast-acting neurotransmitter of inhibitory interneurons [1,2]. Its activity as fast-acting neurotransmitter on nerve cells is mediated by GABA(A) receptor (GABA(A)-R). GABA(A)-R is an ionotropic receptor coupled to chloride ion (Cl^-) channels. The interaction of GABA with GABA(A)-Rs leads to the opening of Cl^- channels and influx of Cl^- in the cells. The entrance of Cl^- inside the cells hyperpolarizes the nerve cells' membrane potential and increases the membrane conductance [3]. The cells become less excitable. Hence, GABA inhibits the transmission of nerve activity. In nerve cells, glutamate decarboxylase (GAD) is the GABA biosynthetic enzyme; GAD catalyzes the decarboxylation of glutamate to GABA

[4,5]. The brain contains two forms of GAD, GAD65 and GAD67. GAD65 is involved in the synthesis of the neurotransmitter pool of GABA, whereas GAD67 is primarily involved in the synthesis of the metabolic pool of GABA [5,6]. High concentration of GABA in nerve endings and GAD are considered landmarks of GABAergic nerve cells; cells that use GABA as neurotransmitter [5,7].

Cerebral plasticity is the dynamic potential of the brain to reorganize itself, during events like ontogeny, learning or following damages [8]. Evidences reveal that GABA is not only a neurotransmitter of inhibitory interneurons. GABA produces excitatory activity on nerve cells on certain situations, as during development. Some glutamatergic excitatory nerve cells may also elicit a GABA phenotype and use GABA as a co-neurotransmitter. Hence, the GABAergic phenotype elicits some form of plasticity.

Excitatory Activity of GABA

During Development and in the Adult Nervous System

In the developing nervous system, GABA has been reported to act as an excitatory neurotransmitter in certain nerve cell populations. GABA depolarizes immature neurons in the developing cerebral cortex [9,10]. In the hippocampus, the granule cells of the dentate gyrus, that project to the pyramidal cells of the *Cornu Ammonis* (CA) region CA3, develop mostly during the first two weeks postnatal [11,12]. During the first week postnatal, GABA exerts a depolarizing activity on the membrane potential of hippocampal neurons of the CA3 region [13-18]. Upon completion of the postnatal maturation of the hippocampus, GABA exerts an inhibitory activity on CA3 pyramidal cells [19]. While most of these observations have been made in the developing brain, GABA has also been reported to depolarize striatal neurons *in vivo* in the adult rat [20]. This shows that GABA acts transiently as an excitatory neurotransmitter during development of the nervous system, and that GABA may also act as an excitatory neurotransmitter in the adult brain.

Circadian Rhythms

The suprachiasmatic nucleus (SCN) is a center for the generation of circadian rhythms in the mammalian nervous system. Cells in the SCN undergo spontaneous changes in their electrical properties between day and night [21]. Particularly, SCN cells show a daily rhythm in the GABA activity; the time of day determines whether GABA acts as an inhibitory or an excitatory transmitter in the SCN. GABA exerts a hyperpolarizing activity on neurons of the SCN during the night and a depolarizing activity during the day [22]. Hence, there is a diurnal change in GABA-signaling in the SCN; GABAergic neurons switch from inhibitory at night to excitatory during the day.

Traumatic Injury

After traumatic brain injury, GABA both synaptically released and exogenously applied exerts a depolarizing activity on neuronal cells surrounding the lesion [23]. The reversal of the role of GABA occurs minutes after trauma and extends for 2-3 weeks after injury. This shows that after trauma, GABA activity switches from inhibitory to excitatory in the lesion area.

In all, in the nervous system GABA elicits a depolarizing activity and acts as an excitatory neurotransmitter, in certain situations.

Reversal of Cl^- Distribution

The activity of the fast acting neurotransmitter GABA is mediated through its interaction with the GABA(A)-R. The GABA(A)-R is coupled to the opening of Cl^- channels. The intracellular concentration of Cl^- is not distributed passively in cells. Chloride ions are transported across the membrane of nerve cells through potassium/chloride ions cotransporters (KCC); Cl^- is transported outward in the cells [24,25]. Upon interaction of GABA with GABA(A)-Rs, the opening of Cl^- channels leads to an influx of Cl^- inside the cells and hyperpolarization of the nerve cells' membrane potential. As consequence, the cells become less excitable. GABA inhibits the transmission of nerve activity.

It is proposed that a reversal in the distribution of Cl^- in nerve cells underlies the switch of GABA activity from hyperpolarizing to depolarizing. During development, circadian rhythm in the SCN and traumatic brain injury, there is an inversion of the Cl^- driving force; Cl^- is transported inward in nerve cells. Hence in these situations, upon interaction of GABA with GABA(A)-Rs, the opening of Cl^- channels leads to an efflux of Cl^- of the cells. This efflux of Cl^- leads to the depolarization of nerve cells' membrane potential and decrease of the membrane conductance. As a consequence, the cells become more excitable. In these situations, GABA acts as an excitatory neurotransmitter and promotes the transmission of nerve activity [9,10,13-18,20,22,23].

The mechanism for the reversal of Cl^- distribution remains to be fully determined. In the rat hippocampus, the expression of an isoform of KCC, KCC2, begins around the first week after birth [26]. The expression of KCC2 correlates with the GABA activity switch from depolarizing to hyperpolarizing and is enough to reverse the cell's distribution of Cl^- inside the cells from high to low. The expression of KCC would underlie the switch of activity of the fast-inhibitory neurotransmitter GABA in the hippocampus from depolarizing to hyperpolarizing [26].

In all, in the nervous system the reversal of the distribution of the Cl^- inside the cells underlies the depolarizing activity of GABA during development, in the adult, during the circadian rhythm and traumatic brain injury.

The function of the depolarizing activity of GABA remains to be fully understood. The depolarizing activity of GABA may lead to an increase in nerve transmission activity. During development, depolarizing activity of GABA onto CA3 pyramidal cells would contribute to synaptic integration and survival of newly generated neuronal cells [27-33]. During traumatic brain injury, it may result in an influx of calcium ions inside the cells, a toxic event leading to cell death [23,34].

GABA Phenotype in Glutamatergic Nerve Cells

Several studies have reported that excitatory glutamatergic nerve cells express a GABA phenotype, *in vitro* and *in vivo*. Among them, glutamatergic striatal neurons expressed GAD immunoreactivity in culture [35]. GAD65 mRNA is expressed in both inhibitory and excitatory hippocampal neurons in culture [36,37], while only a subset of the neuronal cells in culture expresses GAD protein and GABA [38]. CA1 hippocampal pyramidal neurons, a population of glutamatergic excitatory neurons, express GAD65 and GAD67 mRNAs in slice preparations, but no GAD protein or GABA are detected in those cells *in situ* [36-38]. This shows that GAD expression is upregulated *in vitro* in nerve cells that do not normally use GABA as a neurotransmitter. Particularly, in those cells, the translation, but not the transcription, of GAD is induced.

In situ, dentate granule cells, an excitatory glutamatergic population of nerve cells of the hippocampus, express GABA and GAD65 immunoreactivities [39]. Those cells also express low level of GAD65 immunoreactivity and its expression is upregulated in conditions of hyperactivity and during seizures [40-42]. This reveals that some glutamatergic excitatory neurons elicit a dual phenotype, glutamatergic and GABAergic, in the adult brain, particularly hippocampal granule cells [43,44].

These data suggest that, on the one hand, GAD transcription can be upregulated in nerve cells in culture, without these cells using GABA as a neurotransmitter. In the nervous system, GAD expression in nerve cells in considered as marker of GABAergic neurons [5]. This reveals that GAD mRNA expression is not a criterion sufficient to identify a population of nerve cells as GABAergic, particularly *in vitro*.

On the other hand, these data also suggest that glutamatergic excitatory neurons may use GABA as a neurotransmitter *in vivo*. Alternatively, beside its role as a neurotransmitter, GABA may play a metabolic, trophic and neuroprotective role in those cells [45,46]. GABA is synthesized in the cytoplasm of neurons by decarboxylation of Glu by GAD and is metabolized by GABA-aminotransferase to succinic semialdehyde. Succinic semialdehyde is then oxidized to succinate. The conversion of Glu to GABA and subsequently to succinate semialdehyde is known as the GABA shunt. It represents a way for the cells to produce energy from Glu without production of ammonia [45]. GAD may also be use by the cells to produce GABA as trophic support [46] and to reduce the concentration of Glu that in certain condition can be toxic for the cells [34].

In all, the expression of a GABA phenotype in nerve cells may not only signify the use of GABA as a neurotransmitter in those cells, but also its involvement in metabolic, trophic and neuroprotective processes [47]. Interestingly, GAD mRNA expression has been reported in culture without transcription of the protein. A pool of mRNA may provide the cells with the capacity to rapidly synthesize GABA without requiring transcription of the synthetic enzyme. It could be part of the neuron's defense against injuries. The understanding of the mechanism of regulation of GAD transcription and translation may hold cues on the developmental, metabolic, trophic and neuroprotective roles of GABA, versus its role as neurotransmitter, particularly in glutamatergic nerve cells.

CONCLUSION

In the nervous system, different populations of nerve cells are believed to contain either an excitatory or inhibitory fast-acting neurotransmitter, defining excitatory and inhibitory neurons, respectively [48]. In the vertebrate nervous system, Glu is the main excitatory neurotransmitters and GABA the main inhibitory neurotransmitter.

Reports show that GABA may also have transiently a depolarizing activity on nerve cells and thereby act as an excitatory neurotransmitter in certain conditions, as during development, circadian rhythms and traumatic brain injuries. Glutamatergic excitatory nerve cells may also express a GABAergic phenotype. In these cells, GABA may be use as a neurotransmitter. Alternatively, it may play a metabolic, trophic or neuroprotective role. Further investigations are required to determine the functional and physiopathological roles of the excitatory activity of GABA and of the GABA in excitatory nerve cells.

Hence, nerve cells elicit phenotypic plasticity; they may adapt their neurotransmitter phenotype in response to environmental stimuli. The understanding of the mechanisms underlying the phenotype plasticity of neurotransmitters, particularly of GABA, is as important for our understanding of the development of the nervous system, as for our understanding of the physiopathological role of neurotransmitters and the development of new drugs, particularly for the treatment of traumatic brain injuries.

REFERENCES

[1] Ribak CE, Seress L. (1983) Five types of basket cell in the hippocampal dentate gyrus: a combined Golgi and electron microscopic study. *J Neurocytol. 12*, 577-97.

[2] Seress L, Ribak CE. (1983) GABAergic cells in the dentate gyrus appear to be local circuit and projection neurons. *Exp Brain Res. 50*, 173-82.

[3] Sivilotti L, Nistri A. (1991) GABA receptor mechanisms in the central nervous system. *Progress in Neurobiology. 36*, 35-92.

[4] Roberts E, Frankel S. (1950) Aminobutyric acid in brain: its formation from glutamic acid. *J Biol Chem. 187*, 55-63.

[5] Erlander MG, Tillakaratne NJ, Feldblum S, Patel N, Tobin AJ. (1991) Two genes encode distinct glutamate decarboxylases. *Neuron. 7*, 91-100.

[6] Erlander MG, Tobin AJ. (1991) The structural and functional heterogeneity of glutamic acid decarboxylase: a review. *Neurochem Res. 16*, 215-26.

[7] Ribak CE, Vaughn JE, Saito K. (1978) Immunocytochemical localization of glutamic acid decarboxylase in neuronal somata following colchicine inhibition of axonal transport. *Brain Res. 140*, 315-32.

[8] Duffau H. (2006) Brain plasticity: from pathophysiological mechanisms to therapeutic applications. *J Clin Neurosci. 13*, 885-97.

[9] LoTurco JJ, Owens DF, Heath MJ, Davis MB, Kriegstein AR. (1995) GABA and glutamate depolarize cortical progenitor cells and inhibit DNA synthesis. *Neuron. 15*, 1287-98.

[10] Owens DF, Boyce LH, Davis MB, Kriegstein AR. (1996) Excitatory GABA responses in embryonic and neonatal cortical slices demonstrated by gramicidin perforated-patch recordings and calcium imaging. *J Neurosci. 16*, 6414-23.

[11] Gaarskjaer FB. (1986) The organization and development of the hippocampal mossy fiber system. *Brain Res. 396*, 335-57.

[12] Altman J, Bayer SA. (1990) Migration and distribution of two populations of hippocampal granule cell precursors during the perinatal and postnatal periods. *J Comp Neurol. 301*, 365-81.

[13] Ben-Ari Y, Cherubini E, Corradetti R, Gaiarsa JL. (1989) Giant synaptic potentials in immature rat CA3 hippocampal neurones. *J Physiol. 416*, 303-25.

[14] Cherubini E, Rovira C, Gaiarsa JL, Corradetti R, Ben Ari Y. (1990) GABA mediated excitation in immature rat CA3 hippocampal neurons. *Int J Dev Neurosci. 8*, 481-90.

[15] Cherubini E, Gaiarsa JL, Ben-Ari Y. (1991) GABA: an excitatory transmitter in early postnatal life. *Trends Neurosci. 14*, 515-9. Michelson HB, Wong RK. (1991) Excitatory synaptic responses mediated by GABAA receptors in the hippocampus. *Science. 253*, 1420-3.

[16] Ben-Ari Y, Tseeb V, Raggozzino D, Khazipov R, Gaiarsa JL. (1994) Gamma-Aminobutyric acid (GABA): a fast excitatory transmitter which may regulate the development of hippocampal neurones in early postnatal life. *Prog Brain Res. 102*, 261-73.

[17] Khalilov I, Dzhala V, Ben-Ari Y, Khazipov R. (1999) Dual role of GABA in the neonatal rat hippocampus. *Dev Neurosci. 21*, 310-9.

[18] Leinekugel X, Khalilov I, McLean H, Caillard O, Gaiarsa JL, Ben-Ari Y, Khazipov R. (1999) GABA is the principal fast-acting excitatory transmitter in the neonatal brain. *Adv Neurol. 79*, 189-201.

[19] Gaiarsa JL, McLean H, Congar P, Leinekugel X, Khazipov R, Tseeb V, Ben-Ari Y. (1995) Postnatal maturation of gamma-aminobutyric acidA and B-mediated inhibition in the CA3 hippocampal region of the rat. *J Neurobiol. 26*, 339-49.

[20] Mercuri NB, Calabresi P, Stefani A, Stratta F, Bernardi G. (1991) GABA depolarizes neurons in the rat striatum: an in vivo study. *Synapse. 8*, 38-40.

[21] Ko CH, Takahashi JS. (2006) Molecular components of the mammalian circadian clock. *Hum Mol Genet. 15*, R271-7.

[22] Wagner S, Castel M, Gainer H, Yarom Y. (1997) GABA in the mammalian suprachiasmatic nucleus and its role in diurnal rhythmicity. *Nature. 387*, 598-603.

[23] van den Pol AN, Obrietan K, Chen G. (1996) Excitatory actions of GABA after neuronal trauma. *J Neurosci. 16*, 4283-92.

[24] Payne JA, Stevenson TJ, Donaldson LF. (1996) Molecular characterization of a putative K-Cl cotransporter in rat brain. A neuronal-specific isoform. *J Biol Chem. 271*, 16245-52.

[25] Vardi N, Zhang LL, Payne JA, Sterling P. (2000) Evidence that different cation chloride cotransporters in retinal neurons allow opposite responses to GABA. *J Neurosci. 20*, 7657-63.

[26] Rivera C, Voipio J, Payne JA, Ruusuvuori E, Lahtinen H, Lamsa K, Pirvola U, Saarma M, Kaila K. (1999) The K+/Cl- co-transporter KCC2 renders GABA hyperpolarizing during neuronal maturation. *Nature. 397*, 251-5.

[27] Ben-Ari Y, Tseeb V, Raggozzino D, Khazipov R, Gaiarsa JL. (1994) gamma-Aminobutyric acid (GABA): a fast excitatory transmitter which may regulate the development of hippocampal neurones in early postnatal life. *Prog Brain Res. 102*, 261-73.

[28] Katz LC, Shatz CJ. (1996) Synaptic activity and the construction of cortical circuits, *Science. 274*, 1133-8.

[29] Ben-Ari Y, Khazipov R, Leinekugel X, Caillard O, Gaiarsa JL. (1997) GABAA, NMDA and AMPA receptors: a developmentally regulated 'menage a trois'. *Trends Neurosci. 20*, 523-9.

[30] Ben-Ari Y. (2001) Developing networks play a similar melody. *Trends Neurosci. 24*, 353-60.

[31] Owens DF, Kriegstein AR. (2002) Is there more to GABA than synaptic inhibition? *Nat Rev Neurosci. 3*, 715-27.

[32] Ben-Ari Y. (2002) Excitatory actions of gaba during development: the nature of the nurture. *Nat Rev Neurosci. 3*, 728-39.

[33] Gaiarsa JL, Caillard O, Ben-Ari Y. (2002) Long-term plasticity at GABAergic and glycinergic synapses: mechanisms and functional significance. *Trends Neurosci. 25*, 564.

[34] Zipfel GJ, Babcock DJ, Lee JM, Choi DW. (2000) Neuronal apoptosis after CNS injury: the roles of glutamate and calcium. *J Neurotrauma. 17*, 857-69.

[35] Dubinsky JM. (1989) Development of inhibitory synapses among striatal neurons in vitro. *J Neurosci. 9*, 3955-65.

[36] Wilcox KS, Buchhalter J, Dichter MA. (1994) Properties of inhibitory and excitatory synapses between hippocampal neurons in very low density cultures. *Synapse. 18*, 128-51.

[37] Maki R, Robinson MB, Dichter MA. (1994) The glutamate uptake inhibitor L-trans-pyrrolidine-2,4-dicarboxylate depresses excitatory synaptic transmission via a presynaptic mechanism in cultured hippocampal neurons. *J Neurosci. 14*, 6754-62.

[38] Cao Y, Wilcox KS, Martin CE, Rachinsky TL, Eberwine J, Dichter MA. (1996) Presence of mRNA for glutamic acid decarboxylase in both excitatory and inhibitory neurons. *Proc Natl Acad Sci U S A. 93*, 9844-9.

[39] Sandler R, Smith AD. (1991) Coexistence of GABA and glutamate in mossy fiber terminals of the primate hippocampus: an ultrastructural study. *J Comp Neurol. 303*, 177-92.

[40] Houser CR, Esclapez M. (1994) Localization of mRNAs encoding two forms of glutamic acid decarboxylase in the rat hippocampal formation. *Hippocampus. 4*, 530-45.

[41] Schwarzer C, Sperk G. (1995) Hippocampal granule cells express glutamic acid decarboxylase-67 after limbic seizures in the rat. *Neurosci. 69*, 705-9.

[42] Gomez-Lira G, Trillo E, Rami;rez M, Asai M, Sitges M, Gutierrez R. (2002) The Expression of GABA in Mossy Fiber Synaptosomes Coincides with the Seizure-Induced Expression of GABAergic Transmission in the Mossy Fiber Synapse. *Exp Neurol. 177*, 276-83.

[43] Gutierrez R. (203) The GABAergic phenotype of the "glutamatergic" granule cells of the dentate gyrus. *Prog Neurobiol. 71*, 337-58.

[44] Gutierrez R, Romo-Parra H, Maqueda J, Vivar C, Ramirez M, Morales MA, Lamas M. (2003) Plasticity of the GABAergic phenotype of the "glutamatergic" granule cells of the rat dentate gyrus. *J Neurosci. 23*, 5594-8.

[45] Balazs R, Machiyama Y, Hammond BJ, Julian T, Richter D. (1970) The operation of the gamma-aminobutyrate bypath of the tricarboxylic acid cycle in brain tissue in vitro. *Biochem J. 116*, 445-61.

[46] Lipton SA, Kater SB. (1989) Neurotransmitter regulation of neuronal outgrowth, plasticity and survival. *Trends Neurosci. 12*, 265-70.

[47] Waagepetersen HS, Sonnewald U, Schousboe A. (1999) The GABA paradox: multiple roles as metabolite, neurotransmitter, and neurodifferentiative agent. *J Neurochem. 73*, 1335-42.

[48] Roberts E. (1991) Living systems are tonically inhibited, autonomous optimizers, and disinhibition coupled to variability generation is their major organizing principle: inhibitory command-control at levels of membrane, genome, metabolism, brain, and society. *Neurochem Res. 16*, 409-21.

Chapter VII

MOSSY FIBERS AND GABA

ABSTRACT

The granule cells are the nerve cells of the principal layer of the dentate gyrus (DG) of the hippocampus. They are glutamatergic excitatory. Their axons, the mossy fibers (MFs), project to the *Cornu Ammonis* (CA) region CA3, where they establish synaptic connections with dendritic spines of pyramidal cells, in the *stratum lucidum*. The synapses MF-CA3 pyramidal cells elicit unique histological, biochemical and physiopathological features. In 1994, γ-aminobutyric acid (GABA), the main inhibitory neurotransmitter of the nervous system, was detected in MF nerve endings of primates by immunohistochemistry. Glutamate (glutamic acid, Glu) and GABA can be co-released from MF terminals (MFTs) and monosynaptic GABAergic responses can be evoked at the MF-CA3 pyramidal cell synapses by MF activation. The GABA biosynthetic enzyme, glutamate decarboxylase (GAD), is expressed at low level in granule cells, and its expression is upregulated in conditions of hyperactivity and during seizures. CA3 pyramidal cells express GABA receptors and MFTs GABA transporters. In, all GABA is present in MFTs and acts as a neurotransmitter at the MF synapse. The co-existence of two functional neurotransmitters, excitatory and inhibitory, reveals a dual mode of transmission at the MF synapse. This dual mode may underlie unique developmental and physiopathological features of the MF synapse.

INTRODUCTION

The nervous system uses primarily two modes of synaptic transmission, excitatory and inhibitory. These two modes of transmission are believed to be mediated by distinct nerve cell populations, containing excitatory or inhibitory neurotransmitters. In the nervous system, Glu is the main excitatory neurotransmitter and GABA the main inhibitory neurotransmitter [1-5]. In the hippocampus, neurons of the try-synaptic circuit, granule and pyramidal cells, are glutamatergic excitatory, whereas inhibitory interneurons are GABAergic [6-8]. This mode of separation of synaptic activity is at the basis of the functioning of the nervous system as a network; excitatory neuronal cells produce synaptic inputs that stimulate target cells and, in turn, receive inhibitory inputs that govern their excitability [9].

The mossy fibers (MFs) are the axons of the dentate granule cells. The synapses of the MFs are excitatory glutamatergic; they use Glu as their main neurotransmitter [10-12]. The MFs establish synaptic contacts with the spines of CA3 pyramidal cells, in the *stratum lucidum* [13,14]. The synapse MF-CA3 pyramidal cells of MF terminals (MFTs) have a characteristic morphology: they have a large diameter, up to 10 µm, high synaptic vesicles density, mitochondria and a complex morphology, with multiple invaginations and dendritic spines invaginated in the boutons [15,16]. MFTs also contain various other substances, like opioid peptides, trophic factors and zinc [17,22].

In 1991, Sandler and Smith reported the presence of GABA in the synapse MF-CA3 pyramidal cells of monkeys and humans, by immunohistochemistry and electron microscopy [23]. The presence of GABA in MFTs raises the possibility that it may act as a neurotransmitter at the MFTs and that MFTs, that are glutamatergic excitatory, co-release an excitatory neurotransmitter and an inhibitory neurotransmitter, GABA. Further studies have aimed at identifying and characterizing the role of GABA at the MF-CA3 pyramidal cells synapse. The presence of an inhibitory neurotransmitter in an excitatory nerve cell population has profound implications not only for our understanding of the functioning and physiopathology of the MF synapse, but also of the development of the nervous system.

GABA and its Synthetic Enzyme, GAD, in Mossy Fiber Terminals

In 1984, Ottersen and Storm-Mathisen reported immunoreactivity for GABA in the *stratum lucidum* of mouse and rat, in light microscopy [24]. The authors suggested that there was GABA-immunoreactivity within the MF pathway. Others confirmed the presence of GABA-immunoreactivity in the *stratum lucidum* [25] and reported GAD-immunoreactivity in the CA3 region [26]. GAD is the biosynthetic enzyme for GABA [27,28]. Woodson et al. (1989) confirmed the presence of GABA-immunoreactivity in the *hilus* and *stratum lucidum*. Woodson et al. (1989) further reported that GABA-immunoreactivity was not within the granule cells and MF pathway [29]. In 1989, Frotscher reported that MFTs making synaptic contacts with dendrites of GAD immunoreactive cells in the *stratum lucidum* in rat do not contain GAD-immunoreactivity. This study was performed at the ultrastructural level by electron microscopy [30]. The presence of GAD immunoreactivity is a strong argument to characterize a neuronal population as GABAergic [31,32]. It was concluded that MFTs do not contain GABA, and granule cells do not synthesize GABA.

In 1991, Sandler and Smith reported GABA-immunoreactivity in MFTs in the CA3 region of the hippocampus of primates, at the ultrastructural level [23]. Immunoreactivity was detected by immunogold staining, in monkey and human tissues. Large MF terminals in the *stratum lucidum*, with high synaptic vesicles density, mitochondria and dendritic spines invaginated in the boutons, characteristics of MF-CA3 synapses, elicit Glu- and GABA-immunoreactivity. The authors reported weak GAD67- and no GAD65-immunoreactivity in the presynaptic MF nerve endings [23]. This result is in conflict with previous reports showing that there is no GABA- and no GAD-immunoreactivity in the MFTs [29,30]. The co-localization of Glu and GABA in synapse MF-CA3 pyramidal cells suggest that the two amino acids could be co-release by MFTs and that GABA could act as a neurotransmitter at the synapse MF-CA3 pyramidal cells.

In 1994, Taupin et al. reported that Glu and GABA are co-released from fractions enriched in MF synaptosomes (MFSs) [33]. Synaptosomes are "pinched-off" nerve terminals [34,35]. Synaptosome preparations have proven their relevance for studying the physiopathology and pharmacology of ending nerves *in vitro* [36,37]. Taupin et al. (1994) previously reported the isolation and characterization of fractions enriched MFSs. MFSs were isolated by subcellular fractionation on Percoll gradients, from adult rats control and after neonatal irradiation [38]. The authors characterized fractions enriched in MFSs obtained from adult control rats, by their enrichment in synaptosomes eliciting histological biochemical features of MFTs, i.e., a large diameter, with high synaptic vesicle densities, mitochondria and dendritic spines invaginated in the boutons. The authors also estimated the enrichment in MFSs, by assaying dynorphin and zinc, considered markers of MFTs [15-19]. Enrichment in MFSs was confirmed by performing subcellular fractionation from adult rats after neonatal irradiation [38]. Neonatal irradiation of the hippocampal region prevents the development of dentate granule cells in the adult, as the granule cells develop mostly postnatally, during the first two weeks postnatal (figure 1) [39,40]. Subcellular fractionation of the adult hippocampus, after neonatal irradiation, yields fractions depleted in MFSs; fractions obtained from adult rats after neonatal irradiation show a substantial drop in their contents in dynorphin and zinc [38]. This MFS preparation is most useful for studying the MF synapse *ex vivo*.

Previous studies have reported the co-release of Glu and GABA by exocytosis from synaptosome preparations [41,42]. Data from these studies reveal that mechanisms supporting the co-release of Glu and GABA co-exist within individual nerve terminals in the nervous system. Hence, Taupin et al. (1994) investigated the presence and release of Glu, Asp (aspartic acid, Asp) and GABA from MFS preparation [33].

Taupin et al. (1994) characterized fractions enriched in MFSs, from adult rats control and after neonatal irradiation, for their content and ability to release the main amino acid neurotransmitters, Glu, Asp, and GABA [33]. The authors further studied GAD activity in these fractions. No difference in the content of Glu, Asp, and GABA were observed between fractions obtained from adult rats, control and after neonatal irradiation. In contrast, a significant drop in potassium (50 mM, K^+)-evoked calcium ($Ca2^+$)-dependant release of Glu and GABA was observed in fraction enriched in MFSs, obtained from adult rats control versus after neonatal irradiation. No difference in GAD activity was observed between fractions obtained from the adult rats control and after neonatal irradiation [33]. The mechanism of K^+ (50 mM)-evoked release of Glu, Asp, and GABA is not representative of physiological conditions. On the one hand, prolonged K^+-evoked depolarization produces a reversal of the Glu, Asp, and GABA plasma membrane transporters. On the other hand, K^+-evoked depolarization activate voltage-dependent Ca^{2+} channels, allowing Ca^{2+} to reach the interior surface of the cell membrane and trigger fusion and release of vesicularly stored neurotransmitters [43,44]. Hence, K^+-evoked Ca^{2+}-independent release is consistent with reversal of plasma membrane transporters, whereas K^+-evoked Ca^{2+}-dependent release is consistent with exocytosis from vesicularly stored neurotransmitters. The significant drop in K^+-evoked $Ca2^+$-dependant release of Glu and GABA observed in fraction enriched in MFSs, obtained from the adult rats control versus after neonatal irradiation, suggests that Glu and GABA may be co-released from MFTs by exocytosis and that GABA would be present in synaptic vesicles in MFTs. Hence, mechanisms supporting the corelease of Glu and GABA co-exist in MFTs.

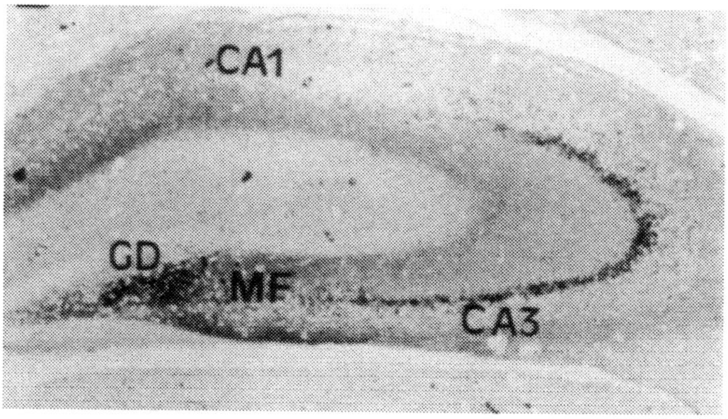

Figure 1. Timm's staining of adult hippocampal section after neonatal irradiation. Rats were submitted to neonatal irradiation of the hippocampal region. Neonatal irradiation of the hippocampal region prevents the development of dentate granule cells in the adult, as the granule cells develop mostly postnatally, during the first two weeks postnatal. Adult rat brains were fixed with paraformaldehyde, processed for histology and Timm's staining. Timm's staining is a histological procedure for staining zinc in tissue section, including the brain. In the hippocampus, the granule cells are the nerve cells of the principal layer of the dentate gyrus (DG), the granule cell layer. Their axons, the mossy fibers (MFs), project to the *Cornu Ammonis* (CA) region CA3 of the hippocampus and establish synaptic contact with the dendritic spines of pyramidal cells. The granule cells and MF terminals are enriched in zinc. In hippocampal sections from adult rats after neonatal irradiation, the absence of Timm's staining in the DG and CA3 region reflects the absence of granule cells in the adult hippocampus. For positive control, refer to chapter 4, figure 3.

Several hypotheses can be raised for the lack of difference observed in Glu, Asp and GABA content, and GAD activity, between fractions enriched in MFSs obtained from adult rats control and those obtained from adult rats after neonatal irradiation. Regarding the lack of difference observed in Glu, Asp and GABA content between fractions enriched in MFSs obtained from the adult rats control and those obtained from adult rats after neonatal irradiation, Glu, Asp and GABA are amino acids present in numerous types of nerve cells and/or glial cells in the brain, and particularly the hippocampus. The lack of differences observed in their content may reflect the contamination from these other cell types in the fractions enriched in MFSs. Regarding the lack of difference observed in GAD activity between fractions enriched in MFSs obtained from the adult rats control and those obtained from the adult rats after neonatal irradiation, several hypotheses can be raised. First, MFTs do not contain GAD, as reported previously [30]. Second, MFTs contain low levels of GAD and the assay used to measure GAD (enzymatic assay) in fractions enriched in MFSs, obtained from adult rats control and those obtained from adult rats after neonatal irradiation, is not sensitive enough to detect such difference. In support of this contention, Sandler and Smith

(1991) reported weak GAD67- and no GAD65-immunoreactivity within the presynaptic MF nerve endings [23]. Third, GAD is present but its enzymatic activity is inhibited and therefore not detectable by the assay. In support of this contention, zinc inhibits GAD activity [37] and is enriched in MFTs [45]. GAD activity may therefore be inhibited in MFTs. However, zinc in MFTs is likely to be in a bound form. The nature of the zinc binding molecules and their distribution in MF synapses remain to be determined. In all, this study does not allow to determine whether MFTs contain GAD, the GABA biosynthetic enzyme. The origin of GABA in MFTs remains to be determined.

The brain contains two forms of GAD, GAD65 and GAD67 [28]. GAD65 is mainly localized in the ending nerves and associated with synthesis of the neurotransmitter pool of GABA. GAD67 in mainly localized in the cell bodies and dendrites and is mainly associated with synthesis of the metabolic pool of GABA [46,47]. Sandler and Smith (1991) reported weak GAD67- and no GAD65-immunoreactivity within the presynaptic MF nerve endings [23]. Therefore, the origin of GABA in MFTs remains to be determined. and several hypotheses can be drawn. GABA could be synthesized by GAD in MFTs. This remains to be demonstrated, particularly as Frotscher (1989) did not detect GAD in MFTs and Sandler and Smith (1991) reported no GAD65-immunoreactivity within MFTs [23,30]. Alternatively, GABA could originate from other metabolic pathways, independent of GAD, from glutamine for example [48,49]. GABA could originate by uptake from the extracellular medium [30]. With regard to this latter hypothesis, there is no evidence that non-GABAergic neurons have the ability to uptake GABA. The presence of GABA transporters is restricted to neurons that synthesize and release GABA, as neurotransmitter, and glial cells [50-52]. Antibodies to neuronal GABA transporter, labels only GABAergic neurons [53]. This shows that GABA membrane transporter is specific of GABAergic neurons. Hence, whether MFTs could uptake GABA from the local environment, without synthesizing it, remains to be demonstrated. It particularly requires identification of GABA membrane transporters in MFTs. In all, the origin of GABA in MFTs remains to be determined.

GABA- and low level of GAD-immunoreactivity in granule cells and MFTs have been reported in rats, mice and monkeys by other groups [54-56], confirming the work by Sandler and Smith (1991) [23]. However, the origin of GABA in MFTs still remains to be resolved. The co-release of Glu and GABA from MFSs suggests that Glu and GABA may be co-released from MFTs and therefore GABA could act as a neurotransmitter at the MFTs [33], a hypothesis that remains to be demonstrated.

GAD Expression is Increased in Granule Cells in Conditions of Hyperactivity and After Seizures

In contrast to control animals, which elicit low levels of GAD, at both protein and mRNA levels, the expression of GAD proteins and mRNAs is increased in rodents in conditions of hyperactivity, like during long-term potentiation and after experimental seizures, after kindling and kainic acid treatment [54-58]. After kainic acid-induced seizures in rats, the expression of GAD67 mRNAs increases transiently in the granule cell layer, 6-24 h after the administration of the drug [54]. The level of GABA is also increased in MFTs after experimental seizures, as reveled by an increase in GABA level in fractions enriched in MFSs isolated from kindled rats [59]. This shows that hyperactivity, and particularly seizures, stimulate the expression of GAD in granule cells and increase the level of GABA in the MFTs. This suggests that GABA may play an important role at the MF synapse during hyperactivity. It may play a role in neurotransmission during hyperactivity, though this remains to be elucidated.

The presence of GABA in MFTs and the GABA synthesizing enzyme, GAD, in granule cells supports a role of GABA in neurotransmission at the MF-CA3 synapse. It remains to demonstrate the functional release, post-synaptic activity and existence of transporters of GABA at the MF-CA3 synapse, order to confirm the role of GABA as a neurotransmitter at the MF-CA3 synapse.

Physiology of the Mossy Fiber Synapse

Walker et al. (2001) reported that monosynaptic GABAergic responses can be evoked at the MF-CA3 pyramidal cell synapse by MF activation, in slices of young guinea pig hippocampus [60]. The synaptic transmission elicits GABAergic responses with characteristics of MF origin; it is not inhibited by antagonists of excitatory amino acid receptors and appears to be GABAergic since it is blocked by picrotoxin, an antagonist of the ionotropic GABA-A receptor [61,62]. This suggests that the monosynaptic GABAergic responses observed on CA3 pyramidal cells is mediated by the stimulation of the MFs themselves. There are other alternatives for this observation, like the co-stimulation of MFs with GABAergic fibers of a projecting inhibitory pathway that would run in parallel with the MFs [29] or with sprouted interneurons [63]. However, the mediation by the stimulation of the MFs themselves is the most likely explanation for the origin of the monosynaptic GABAergic responses observed at the MF-CA3 pyramidal cell synapse in guinea pig.

This study provides the first evidence of a physiological role of GABA present in MFTs. It suggests that the GABAergic responses evoked at the MF-CA3 pyramidal cell synapse is mediated by the release of GABA from the MFTs. It further supports the hypothesis that GABA present in MFTs acts as a neurotransmitter at the MF-CA3 pyramidal cell synapse.

In rat, in contrast to guinea pig, GABAergic transmission at MF-CA3 pyramidal cell synapses is detected after seizures, but not in control conditions [64]. In rat, GABAergic transmission at the MFTs would be activity- and protein synthesis-dependent [65-67]. This would go inline with histological studies showing that the content of GABA and GAD activity in granule cells and MFTs are increased in conditions of hyperactivity and after seizures [54-59]. However, others have confirmed the observations reported by Walker et al. (2001) that monosynaptic GABAergic responses at the MF-CA3 pyramidal cell synapse is observed in naïve animals, including rodents [68].

In all, these results show that the MFTs use GABA as a neurotransmitter and elicit GABAergic inhibitory transmission at the MF-CA3 pyramidal cell synapse, an excitatory glutamatergic synapse. It suggests the existence of GABA receptors on post-synaptic membranes of CA3 pyramidal cells. The release of an inhibitory neurotransmitter in an excitatory glutamatergic synapse also raises the question of the function of GABA at the

MFTs. It remains to demonstrate i) that GABA acts on post-synaptic receptors at the MF-CA3 pyramidal cells synapse and ii) that MFTs express GABA plasma membrane and vesicular transporters, to inactivate GABA signaling and for synaptic release of GABA.

GABA Receptors and Transporters at the Mossy Fiber Synapse

In vitro, the application of GABA onto CA3 pyramidal cells produces a hyperpolarization [69]. This suggests that CA3 pyramidal cells express GABA receptors. Two types of receptors mediate the activity of GABA on nerve cells; GABA receptor type A and B, GABA-(A)R and GABA-(B)R. GABA-(A)R is a ionotropic receptor. GABA-(A)R mediates fast GABAergic transmission, whereas GABA-(B)R is a metabotropic receptor [70,71]. GABA-(A)R is coupled to a chloride-permeable ion channel [62,71]. Synaptically released GABA activates post-synaptic GABA-(A)Rs. This leads to the opening of chloride-permeable ion channels, the entrance of chloride ions inside the cells and hyperpolarization of the post-synaptic membrane. Hyperpolarization increases the membrane conductance. This inhibits the transmission of nerve activity by making nerve cells less responsive to excitatory input.

The GABA-(A)R subunit (g3) is expressed in the *stratum lucidum*, region where the MF projections establish synaptic contacts with the dendritic spines of CA3 pyramidal cells [72]. Electron microscopy studies reveal co-expression of GABA-(A)Rs and Glu receptors (GluRs) at the MF synapses [68]. In all, GABA-(A)Rs may co-exist with GluRs in post-synaptic CA3 pyramidal cells and mediate the GABA synaptic activity originating from the granule cells and MFTs.

GABA is transported inside the cells by a transporter, the plasma membrane GABA transporter (GAT). GAT uses energy provided by the transmembrane sodium gradient to transport GABA inside the cells. Two types of plasma membrane GABA transporters have been identified, GAT-1 and GAT-2 [73-75]. In the central nervous system (CNS), GAT is expressed in neurons that synthesize and release GABA, and in glial cells [74-76]. GABA is transported inside synaptic vesicles by transporters, the vesicular GABA transporters (VGAT) [76,77].

In the hippocampus, GAT-1 is primarily expressed by interneurons and glial cells [78]. Granule cells also express GAT-1 mRNAs and the level of expression of GAT-1 mRNAs is enhanced in the DG following kindled seizures in rat [79]. MFSs uptake GABA, an activity inhibited by the selective GABA uptake blocker, nipecotic acid [59]. Finally, VGAT mRNAs are expressed in the DG and in MFTs in control rats, and their expression is enhanced in MFTs after seizures [80]. In all, these data show that both GAT and VGAT are presents on granule cells and MFs, and may account for the transport of GABA inside MFTs and synaptic vesicles. This further supports that the role of GABA presents in MFTs as a neurotransmitter at the MF-CA3 pyramidal cell synapse.

SIGNIFICANCE OF THE PRESENCE OF GABA IN MOSSY FIBER TERMINALS

MFTs contain GABA, an inhibitory neurotransmitter [23]. GAD, GAT and VGAT are expressed in granule cells and MFTs. GABA-(A)Rs are expressed in the *stratum lucidum*, region of projection of the MFs in the CA3 hippocampal subfield [54-58]. This shows that all the components necessary for GABA synaptic transmission at the MF synapse are presents. Evidences further suggest that GABA is co-released with Glu from the MFTs [33] and show the synapse MF-CA3 pyramidal cells elicits electrophysiological characteristic of inhibitory monosynaptic GABA transmission, with characteristics of MF origin [60].

These data support the role of GABA as a neurotransmitter at the MF-CA3 pyramidal cell synapse and that Glu and GABA are co-released from MFTs. In support to this contention, Bergersen et al. (2003) using electron microscopy and high resolution immunogold cytochemistry showed that Glu and GABA are co-localized within most MFTs, and that Glu and GABA are associated with synaptic vesicles in MFTs, in rat [68]. Therefore, the MF synapse represents a model of "dual" synapse, with two "fast-acting" neurotransmitters, Glu and GABA, respectively excitatory and inhibitory neurotransmitters [81,82]. This raises the question of the mechanism of co-release of the neurotransmitters and the function of GABA at the MF-CA3 pyramidal cell synapse.

In the nervous system, excitatory and inhibitory transmissions are believed to be carried out by separate populations of nerve cells [9]. In the nervous system, and particularly the hippocampus, Glu is the main excitatory neurotransmitters and GABA the main inhibitory neurotransmitter. In the hippocampus, granule and pyramidal cells use Glu as neurotransmitter, whereas inhibitory interneurons use GABA as neurotransmitter [1-7]. The co-localization of an excitatory, Glu, and inhibitory, GABA, neurotransmitter in the MF synapse suggests that the functioning of the MF synapse involve complex regulatory processes and the mechanisms underlying the co- release of Glu and GABA at the MF synapse is likely to be tightly regulated. Future studies will aim at investigating the mechanism of co-release of Glu and GABA at the MFTs. Particularly, future studies will aim at identifying the ratio and kinetic of release of Glu versus GABA at the MFTs, in different experimental conditions, and at characterizing the cellular and molecular mechanisms underlying the co-release of Glu and GABA at the MFTs.

The hippocampal formation is a critical area in the pathology of epilepsy [83]. It is proposed that the DG may function as a gate, controlling the propagation of seizures [84,85]. Granule cells would regulate the throughput of epileptiform activity transiting through the hippocampal formation [86]. GABA and GABA-mediated inhibition are known to regulate neuronal excitability, and to have an anticonvulsant activity [87].

It is proposed that GABA released from MFTs could contribute to a protective role against generation of spontaneous seizures in the hippocampus. This by reducing granule cells hyperactivity during seizures [88]. In support to this contention, increase in GABA synthesis and release from MFTs, during epileptic seizures, may represent an attempt by the nervous system to reduce the Glu over-excitation and toxicity on CA3 pyramidal cells, and return to a normal state [54-59]. GABA may modulate granule cells hyperactivity during seizures either directly by acting through GABA-A(R)s on CA3 pyramidal cells or by acting on presynaptic GABA(B)-Rs. In that latter model, GABA-mediated autoreceptors at MF terminals could represent a further level of modulation of transmission, to prevent over-excitation of the post-synaptic neurons. The protective role of GABA released by MFTs against the generation of spontaneous seizures in the hippocampus remains to be validated. The mechanism of action and role of GABA as a neurotransmitter at the MF synapse, in the physiopathology of the MF synapse, remain to be determined as well.

Conclusion

In the nervous system, excitatory and inhibitory transmissions are believed to be carried out by separate populations of nerve cells. In the hippocampus, neurons of the tri-synaptic circuit, granule and pyramidal cells, are glutamatergic excitatory, whereas inhibitory interneurons are GABAergic. Evidences reveal that dentate granule cells and MFs elicit a dual phenotype; they contain and use GABA as a neurotransmitter. The presence of excitatory and inhibitory neurotransmitters in the MF synapse not only raises the question of the mechanism of action of these neurotransmitters and its functional significance, but it also raises the issue of identifying and defining nerve cell phenotypes, and particularly GABAergic phenotypes.

In the nervous system, nerve cells are defined according to their main "fast-acting" neurotransmitter. Since GABA is synthesized in the cytoplasm of neurons that are GABAergic, the detection of GAD, the GABA synthesizing enzyme, is a criterion well accepted to identify a population of nerve cells as using GABA as neurotransmitter. The granule cells express low levels of GAD that are barely detectable by immunohistochemistry and *in situ* hybridization, in control animals. The lack of detection of GAD mRNAs in granule cells, particularly, mandates caution when using GAD mRNA detection for identifying GABAergic nerve cells. Low levels of GAD mRNAs may prevent its detection, though nerve cells may use GABA as a neurotransmitter -like granule cells-. Therefore, multiple investigations may be needed to be carried out to identify a GABAergic phenotype.

It is proposed that the co-release of Glu and GABA at the MFTs may contribute to a protective role against generation of spontaneous seizures in the hippocampus. Further studies will aim at investigating the role of GABA in MFTs and the mechanism underlying its physiopathological activity.

Acknowledgments

Chapter 7, figure 1, is reprinted, with permission, from *J Neurochem*, Vol 62, Taupin P, Zini S, Cesselin F, Ben-Ari Y, Roisin MP, Subcellular fractionation on Percoll gradient of mossy fiber synaptosomes: morphological and biochemical characterization in control and degranulated rat hippocampus, Pages 1586-95, Copyright (1994), Wiley-Blackwell, Inc.

REFERENCES

[1] Curtis DR, Johnston GA. (1974) Amino acid transmitters in the mammalian central nervous system. *Ergeb Physiol. 69*, 97-188.

[2] Ribak CE, Seress L. (1983) Five types of basket cell in the hippocampal dentate gyrus: a combined Golgi and electron microscopic study. *J Neurocytol. 12*, 577-97.

[3] Seress L, Ribak CE. (1983) GABAergic cells in the dentate gyrus appear to be local circuit and projection neurons. *Exp Brain Res. 50*, 173-82.

[4] Watkins JC. (2000) l-glutamate as a central neurotransmitter: looking back. *Biochem Soc Trans. 28*, 297-309.

[5] Fonnum F. (1984) Glutamate: a neurotransmitter in mammalian brain. *J Neurochem. 42*, 1-11.

[6] Andersen P, Bliss TV, Lomo T, Olsen LI, Skrede KK. (1969) Lamellar organization of hippocampal excitatory pathways. *Acta Physiol Scand. 76*, 4A-5A.

[7] Lambert JD, Jones RS, Andreasen M, Jensen MS, Heinemann U. (1989) The role of excitatory amino acids in synaptic transmission in the hippocampus. *Comp Biochem Physiol A. 93*, 195-201.

[8] McBain CJ, Freund TF, Mody I. (1999) Glutamatergic synapses onto hippocampal interneurons: precision timing without lasting plasticity. *Trends Neurosci. 22*, 228-35.

[9] Roberts E. (1991) Living systems are tonically inhibited, autonomous optimizers, and disinhibition coupled to variability generation is their major organizing principle: inhibitory command-control at levels of membrane, genome, metabolism, brain, and society. *Neurochem Res. 16*, 409-21.

[10] Crawford I, Connor J. (1973) Localization and release of glutamic acid in relation to the hippocampal mossy fiber pathway. *Nature. 244*, 442-3.

[11] Storm-Mathisen J, Leknes AK, Bore AT, Vaaland JL, Edminson P, Haug FS, Ottersen OP. (1983) First visualization of glutamate and GABA in neurones by immunochemistry. *Nature. 301*, 517-20.

[12] Langdon RB, Johnson JW, Barrionuevo G. (1993) Asynchrony of mossy fibre inputs and excitatory postsynaptic currents in rat hippocampus. *J Physiol. 472*, 157-76.

[13] Blackstad TW, Kjaerheim A. (1961) Special axo-dendritic synapses in the hippocampal cortex: electron and light microscopic studies on the layer of the mossy fibers. *J. Comp. Neurol. 117*, 133-59.

[14] Gaarskjaer FB. (1986) The organization and development of the hippocampal mossy fiber system. *Brain Res. 396*, 335-57.

[15] Hamlyn LH. (1962) The fine structure of the mossy fiber endings in the hippocampus of the rabbit. *J. Anat. (London). 96*, 112-20.

[16] Niklowitz W. (1966) Elektronenmikroskopische untersuchungen am ammonshorn. *Zeitschrift für Zellforschung. 75*, 485-500.

[17] McLardy T. (1962) Zinc enzymes and the hippocampal mossy fibre system. *Nature. 194*, 300-2.

[18] Haug FMS. (1967) Electron microscopical localization of the zinc in hippocampal mossy fiber synapses by a modified sulfide silver procedure. *Histochimie. 8*, 355-68.

[19] McGinty JF, Henriksen SJ, Goldstein A, Terenius L, Bloom FE. (1983) Dynorphin is contained within hippocampal mossy fibers: immunochemical alterations after kainic acid administration and colchicine induced neurotoxicity. *Proc Natl Acad Sci U S A. 80*, 589-93.

[20] Friedman WJ, Ernfors P, Persson H. (1991) Transient and persistent expression of NT-3/HDNF mRNA in the rat brain during postnatal development. *J Neurosci. 11*, 1577-84.

[21] Taupin P, Roisin MP, Ben-Ari Y, Barbin G. (1994) A fraction enriched in rat hippocampal mossy fibre synaptosomes contains trophic activities. *Neuroreport. 5*, 1353-5.

[22] Vigers AJ, Baquet ZC, Jones KR. (2000) Expression of neurotrophin-3 in the mouse forebrain: insights from a targeted LacZ reporter. *J Comp Neurol. 416*, 398-415.

[23] Sandler R, Smith AD. (1991) Coexistence of GABA and glutamate in mossy fiber terminals of the primate hippocampus: an ultrastructural study. *J Comp Neurol. 303*, 177-92.

[24] Ottersen OP, Storm-Mathisen J. (1984) Glutamate- and GABA-containing neurons in the mouse and rat brain, as demonstrated with a new immunocytochemical technique. *J Comp Neurol. 229*, 374-92.

[25] Gamrani H, Onteniente B, Seguela P, Geffard M, Calas A. (1986) Gamma-aminobutyric acid -immunoreactivity in the rat hippocampus. A light and electron microscopic study with anti-GABA antibodies. *Brain Res. 364*, 30-8.

[26] Babb TL, Pretorius JK, Kupfer WR, Brown WJ. (1988) Distribution of glutamate-decarboxylase immuno-reactive neurons and synapses in rat and monkey hippocampus: light and electron microscopy. *J Comp Neurol. 278*, 121-38.

[27] Roberts E, Frankel S. (1950) Aminobutyric acid in brain: its formation from glutamic acid. *J Biol Chem. 187*, 55-63.

[28] Erlander MG, Tillakaratne NJ, Feldblum S, Patel N, Tobin AJ. (1991) Two genes encode distinct glutamate decarboxylases. *Neuron. 7*, 91-100.

[29] Woodson W, Nitecka L, Ben-Ari Y. (1989) Organization of the GABAergic system in the rat hippocampal formation: a quantitative immunocytochemical study. *J Comp Neurol. 280*, 254-71.

[30] Frotscher M. (1989) Mossy fiber synapses on glutamate decarboxylase-immunoreactive neurons: evidence for feed-forward inhibition in the CA3 region of the hippocampus. *Exp Brain Res. 75*, 441-5.

[31] Ribak CE, Vaughn JE, Saito K. (1978) Immunocytochemical localization of glutamic acid decarboxylase in neuronal somata following colchicine inhibition of axonal transport. *Brain Res. 140*, 315-32.

[32] Erlander MG, Tobin AJ. (1991) The structural and functional heterogeneity of glutamic acid decarboxylase: a review. *Neurochem Res. 16*, 215-26.

[33] Taupin P, Ben-Ari Y, Roisin MP. (1994) Subcellular fractionation on Percoll gradient of mossy fiber synaptosomes: evoked release of glutamate, GABA, aspartate and glutamate decarboxylase activity in control and degranulated rat hippocampus. *Brain Res. 644*, 313-21.

[34] De Robertis E, Pellegrino De Iraldi A, Rodriguez De Lorez Arnaiz G, Gomez J. (1961) On the isolation of nerve endings and synaptic vesicles. *J Biophys Biochem Cytol. 9*, 229-35.

[35] Gray EG, Whittaker VP. (1962) The isolation of nerve endings from brain: an electron-microscopic study of cell fragments derived by homogenization and centrifugation. *J Anat (Lond.). 96*, 79-87.

[36] Whittaker VP. (1993) Thirty years of synaptosome research. *J Neurocytol. 22*, 735-42.

[37] Raiteri L, Raiteri M. (2000) Synaptosomes still viable after 25 years of superfusion. *Neurochem Res. 25*, 1265-74.

[38] Taupin P, Zini S, Cesselin F, Ben-Ari Y, Roisin MP. (1994) Subcellular fractionation on Percoll gradient of mossy fiber synaptosomes: morphological and biochemical characterization in control and degranulated rat hippocampus. *J Neurochem. 62*, 1586-95.

[39] Bayer SA, Peters PJ. (1977) A method for x-irradiating selected brain regions in infant rats. *Brain Res Bull. 2*, 153-6.

[40] Represa A, Dessi F, Beaudoin M, Ben-Ari Y. (1991) Effects of neonatal gamma-ray irradiation on rat hippocampus--I. Postnatal maturation of hippocampal cells. *Neurosci. 42*, 137-50.

[41] Sihra TS, Nicholls DG. (1987) 4-Aminobutyrate can be released exocytotically from guinea-pig cerebral cortical synaptosomes. *J Neurochem. 49*, 261-7.

[42] Belhage B, Hansen GH, Schousboe A. (1993) Depolarization by K+ and glutamate activates different neurotransmitter release mechanisms in GABAergic neurons: vesicular versus non-vesicular release of GABA. *Neurosci. 54*, 1019-34.

[43] Haycock JW, Levy WB, Denner LA, Cotman CW. (1978) Effects of elevated [K+]O on the release of neurotransmitters from cortical synaptosomes: efflux or secretion? *J Neurochem. 30*, 1113-25.

[44] Bernath S, Zigmond MJ. (1988) Characterization of [3H] GABA release from striatal slices: evidence for a calcium-independent process via the GABA uptake system. *Neurosci. 27*, 563-70.

[45] Wu JY, Roberts E. (1974) Properties of brain L-glutamate decarboxylase: inhibition studies. *J Neurochem. 23*, 759-67.

[46] Kaufman DL, Houser CR, Tobin AJ. (1991) Two forms of the gamma-aminobutyric acid synthetic enzyme glutamate decarboxylase have distinct intraneuronal distributions and cofactor interactions. *J Neurochem. 56*, 720-3.

[47] Waagepetersen HS, Sonnewald U, Gegelashvili G, Larsson OM, Schousboe A. (2001) Metabolic distinction between vesicular and cytosolic GABA in cultured GABAergic neurons using 13C magnetic resonance spectroscopy. *J Neurosci Res. 63*, 347-55.

[48] Reubi JC, Van Der Berg C, Cuénod M. (1978) Glutamine as precursor for the GABA and glutamate transmitter pools. *Neurosci Letters. 10*, 171-4.

[49] Martin DL, Rimvall K. (1993) Regulation of gamma-aminobutyric acid synthesis in the brain. *J Neurochem. 60*, 395-407.

[50] Iversen LL, Kelly JS. (1975) Uptake and metabolism of gamma-aminobutyric acid by neurones and glial cells. *Biochem Pharmacol. 24*, 933-8.

[51] Radian R, Ottersen OP, Storm-Mathisen J, Castel M, Kanner BI. (1990) Immunocytochemical localization of the GABA transporter in rat brain. *J Neurosci. 10*, 1319-30.

[52] Ribak CE, Tong WM, Brecha NC. (1996) GABA plasma membrane transporters, GAT-1 and GAT-3, display different distributions in the rat hippocampus. *J Comp Neurol. 367*, 595-606.

[53] Augood SJ, Herbison AE, Emson PC. (1995) Localization of GAT-1 GABA transporter mRNA in rat striatum: cellular coexpression with GAD67 mRNA, GAD67 immunoreactivity, and parvalbumin mRNA. *J Neurosci. 15*, 865-74.

[54] Schwarzer C, Sperk G. (1995) Hippocampal granule cells express glutamic acid decarboxylase-67 after limbic seizures in the rat. *Neurosci. 69*, 705-9.

[55] Lehmann H, Ebert U, Loscher W. (1996) Immunocytochemical localization of GABA immunoreactivity in dentate granule cells of normal and kindled rats. *Neurosci Lett. 212*, 41-44.

[56] Sloviter RS, Dichter MA, Rachinsky TL, Dean E, Goodman JH, Sollas AL, Martin DL. (1996) Basal expression and induction of glutamate decarboxylase and GABA in excitatory granule cells of the rat and monkey hippocampal dentate gyrus. *J Comp Neurol. 373*, 593-618.

[57] Houser CR, Esclapez M. (1994) Localization of mRNAs encoding two forms of glutamic acid decarboxylase in the rat hippocampal formation. *Hippocampus. 4*, 530-45.

[58] Makiura Y, Suzuki F, Chevalier E, Onteniente B. (1999) Excitatory granule cells of the dentate gyrus exhibit a double inhibitory neurochemical content after intrahippocampal administration of kainate in adult mice. *Exp Neurol. 159*, 73-83.

[59] Gomez-Lira G, Trillo E, Ramirez M, Asai M, Sitges M, Gutierrez R. (2002) The Expression of GABA in Mossy Fiber Synaptosomes Coincides with the Seizure-Induced Expression of GABAergic Transmission in the Mossy Fiber Synapse. *Exp Neurol. 177*, 276-83.

[60] Walker MC, Ruiz A, Kullmann DM. (2001) Monosynaptic GABAergic signaling from dentate to CA3 with a pharmacological and physiological profile typical of mossy fiber synapses. *Neuron. 29*, 703-15.

[61] Andreasen M, Lambert JD, Jensen MS. (1989) Effects of new non-N-methyl-D-aspartate antagonists on synaptic transmission in the in vitro rat hippocampus. *J Physiol. 414*, 317-36.

[62] Mohler H. (2006) GABA(A) receptor diversity and pharmacology. *Cell Tissue Res. 326*, 505-16.

[63] Davenport CJ, Brown WJ, Babb TL. (1990) Sprouting of GABAergic and mossy fiber axons in dentate gyrus following intrahippocampal kainate in the rat. *Exp Neurol. 109*, 180-90.

[64] Gutierrez R. (2000) Seizures induce simultaneous GABAergic and glutamatergic transmission in the dentate gyrus-CA3 system. *J Neurophysiol. 84*, 3088-90.

[65] Gutierrez R, Heinemann U. (2001) Kindling induces transient fast inhibition in the dentate gyrus--CA3 projection. *Eur J Neurosci. 13*, 1371-9.

[66] Gutierrez R. (2002) Activity-dependent expression of simultaneous glutamatergic and GABAergic neurotransmission from the mossy fibers in vitro. *J Neurophysiol. 87*, 2562-70.

[67] Romo-Parra H, Vivar C, Maqueda J, Morales MA, Gutierrez R. (2003) Activity-dependent induction of multitransmitter signaling onto pyramidal cells and interneurons of hippocampal area CA3. *J Neurophysiol. 89*, 3155-67.

[68] Bergersen L, Ruiz A, Bjaalie JG, Kullmann DM, Gundersen V. (2003) GABA and GABAA receptors at hippocampal mossy fibre synapses. *Eur J Neurosci. 18*, 931-41.

[69] Janigro D, Schwartzkroin PA. (1988) Effects of GABA on CA3 pyramidal cell dendrites in rabbit hippocampal slices. *Brain Res. 453*, 265-74.

[70] Bowery NG, Hudson AL, Price GW. (1987) GABA-A and GABA-B receptor site distribution in the rat central nervous system. *Neurosci. 20*, 365-33.

[71] Sivilotti L, Nistri A. (1991) GABA receptor mechanisms in the central nervous system. *Progress in Neurobiology. 36*, 35-92.

[72] Sperk G, Schwarzer C, Tsunashima K, Fuchs K, Sieghart W. (1997) GABA(A) receptor subunits in the rat hippocampus I: immunocytochemical distribution of 13 subunits. *Neurosci. 80*, 987-1000.

[73] Iversen LL, Kelly JS. (1975) Uptake and metabolism of gamma-aminobutyric acid by neurones and glial cells. *Biochem Pharmacol. 24*, 933-8.

[74] Radian R, Ottersen OP, Storm-Mathisen J, Castel M, Kanner BI. (1990) Immunocytochemical localization of the GABA transporter in rat brain. *J Neurosci. 10*, 1319-30.

[75] Ribak CE, Tong WM, Brecha NC. (1996) GABA plasma membrane transporters, GAT-1 and GAT-3, display different distributions in the rat hippocampus. *J Comp Neurol. 367*, 595-606.

[76] McIntire SL, Reimer RJ, Schuske K, Edwards RH, Jorgensen EM. (1997) Identification and characterization of the vesicular GABA transporter. *Nature. 389*, 870-6.

[77] Sagne C, El Mestikawy S, Isambert MF, Hamon M, Henry JP, Giros B, Gasnier B. (1997) Cloning of a functional vesicular GABA and glycine transporter by screening of genome databases. *FEBS Lett. 417*, 177-83.

[78] Frahm C, Engel D, Piechotta A, Heinemann U, Draguhn A. (2000) Presence of gamma-aminobutyric acid transporter mRNA in interneurons and principal cells of rat hippocampus. *Neurosci Lett. 288*, 175-8.

[79] Hirao T, Morimoto K, Yamamoto Y, Watanabe T, Sato H, Sato K, Sato S, Yamada N, Tanaka K, Suwaki H. (1998) Time-dependent and regional expression of GABA transporter mRNAs following amygdala-kindled seizures in rats. *Brain Res Mol Brain Res. 54*, 49-55.

[80] Lamas M, Gomez-Lira G, Gutierrez R. (2001) Vesicular GABA transporter mRNA expression in the dentate gyrus and in mossy fiber synaptosomes. *Brain Res Mol Brain Res. 93*, 209-14.

[81] Gutierrez R. (203) The GABAergic phenotype of the "glutamatergic" granule cells of the dentate gyrus. *Prog Neurobiol. 71*, 337-58.

[82] Gutierrez R, Romo-Parra H, Maqueda J, Vivar C, Ramirez M, Morales MA, Lamas M. (2003) Plasticity of the GABAergic phenotype of the "glutamatergic" granule cells of the rat dentate gyrus. *J Neurosci. 23*, 5594-8.

[83] Thom M. (2004) Recent advances in the neuropathology of focal lesions in epilepsy. *Expert Rev Neurother. 4*, 973-84.

[84] Collins RC, Tearse RG, Lothman EW. (1983) Functional anatomy of limbic seizures: focal discharges from medial entorhinal cortex in rat. *Brain Res. 280*, 25-40.

[85] Heinemann U, Beck H, Dreier JP, Ficker E, Stabel J, Zhang CL. (1992) The dentate gyrus as a regulated gate for the propagation of epileptiform activity. *Epilepsy Res Suppl. 7*, 273-80.

[86] Sloviter RS. (1991) Feedforward and feedback inhibition of hippocampal principal cell activity evoked by perforant path stimulation: GABA-mediated mechanisms that regulate excitability in vivo. *Hippocampus. 1*, 31-40.

[87] Meldrum BS, Rogawski MA. (2007) Molecular targets for antiepileptic drug development. *Neurotherapeutics. 4*, 18-61.

[88] Gutierrez R, Heinemann U. (2006) Co-existence of GABA and Glu in the hippocampal granule cells: implications for epilepsy. *Curr Top Med Chem. 6*, 975-8.

Chapter VIII

DEVELOPMENT OF THE HIPPOCAMPUS

ABSTRACT

The development of the mammalian nervous system initiates prenatally, with most nerve cells born before birth, whereas the process of maturation of the nervous system, gliogenesis and myelination, continue long -decades- after birth. In the hippocampus, the development of granule and pyramidal cells follows different patterns. The development of the *Cornu Ammonis* (CA) initiates in the prenatal period, with most pyramidal cells born prenatally. The maturation process of the CA extends until 2-3 weeks after birth. Contrary to other brain areas, most of the granule cells of the dentate gyrus (DG) are born postnatally, during the first two weeks of life. Their axons, the mossy fibers (MFs), have mainly a postnatal development. The MF synapses establish connections with dendritic spines of pyramidal cells of the CA3 region, in the *stratum lucidum*, coincidently to the appearance of dendritic spines on the pyramidal cells of CA3 around the second week postnatal. During the postnatal period, GABA originating from hilar and CA3 interneurons of the hippocampus would exert a depolarizing activity onto CA3 pyramidal cells. During the postnatal period, granule cells also express transiently a GABAergic excitatory phenotype. The GABA depolarizing activity onto CA3 pyramidal cells and the expression of a GABAergic excitatory phenotype by granule cells, an excitatory glutamatergic population of nerve cells, raise the question of their physiological significances and roles during development.

DEVELOPMENT OF THE HIPPOCAMPAL SUBFIELDS OF THE *CORNU AMMONIS*

The development of the CA initiates in the prenatal period. In mice, neural progenitor cells at the origin of the hippocampal pyramidal cells are born at embryonic (E) day 10.5 [1]. The period of gestation is 19-20 days for housed mice, versus 21-24 days for rats. Neural progenitor cells at the origin of the hippocampal pyramidal cells derive from neural stem cells originating from the ventricular zone [1].

By day E 14.5, most of these progenitor cells have migrated to their final presumptive position to form a detectable cortical plate, where they will give rise to pyramidal cells at the origin of the CA [2,3]. At day E 14.5, pyramidal cells in the first presumptive field of the CA region, the region CA3, express the kainate receptor (KA1). A day later, at E 15.5, pyramidal cells of the presumptive region CA1 express the transcription factor SCIP [4-7]. In rodents, most of the pyramidal cells of the CA regions are generated between the embryonic days 15 and 19, from neural progenitor cells.

The development of the CA subfields into their final states will extend into the postnatal period, until 2-3 weeks after birth [4-7]. Particularly, the dendritic spines of the pyramidal cells of CA3 appear around the second week postnatal [4-7].

The early stages of development of the CA follow primarily a poles-inward pattern, in which cells at the poles of the hippocampus are born first, followed by cells in the middle of the hippocampal region.

The CA regions acquire their specifications early in development, as demonstrated by removing the embryonic CA from its normal environment. Embryonic CA regions isolated, from the developing brain and maintained *in vitro*, develop autonomously a range of mature features specific of CA, without ongoing cues from outside the hippocampus or even from other hippocampal fields [8]. It is proposed that extrinsic innervations and environment may provide early patterning cues that initially subdivide the embryonic CA into its presumptive fields.

In all, the development of the CA occurs during the embryonic development, with the hippocampal CA regions individualized, as early as the migration of the precursor cells of pyramidal cells is completed. The CA regions acquire then very early in development their specification and the maturation of CA fields occurs primarily in a poles-inward pattern, a process that is completed postnatally.

Dentate Gyrus

Granule Cells

The development of granule and pyramidal cells of the hippocampus follows different patterns. Whereas the pyramidal cells of the CA regions, as most other brain nerve cells, are born in the prenatal period, the genesis of granule cells of the DG occurs mostly after birth, during the first two weeks postnatal [9,10].

The first precursor cells of the dentate granule cells are generated at the same time as the precursor cells of the CA3 pyramidal cells and their generation extends beyond birth [11]. About 15% of the granule cells are born before birth, but most of them (70%) are born during the first two weeks of life and 15% after the 16 day postnatal (PN) in mice [1,13]. Newly born granule cells that lie in the inner portion of the granule cells layer may express markers of the GABAergic phenotype [10].

Mossy Fibers

The mossy fibers (MFs), the axons of the granule cells, have mainly a postnatal development [9-12]. The MF synapses establish connections with dendrites of pyramidal cells of the CA3 region, in the *stratum lucidum*. The development of the MF synapses with CA3 pyramidal cells operates in three steps.

During the first phase in rodent, between day PN 3 and PN 9, the growth cones of the granule cells reach the *stratum lucidum* of the CA3 region. The MF ending nerves establish the first synaptic contacts, both symmetrical and asymmetrical, with dendrites of CA3 pyramidal cells. During that time, the MF ending nerves increase in size. At day PN 9, the MF synapses begin their process of invagination of the dendritic spines of the CA3 pyramidal cells.

During the second phase, between day PN 10 and PN 14, the invaginations are becoming more complex, with an increase in the density of synaptic vesicles in the MF endings. Concomitantly appears dendritic spines on CA3 pyramidal cells [4-7].

During the third phase from day PN 14, the MF synapses complete their maturation. Particularly, the process of invagination of CA3 dendritic spines by the MF terminals progresses, with an increase in the number of symmetrical and asymmetrical contacts at the synapse MF-CA3 pyramidal cells. By day PN 21, the MF endings reache their fully mature aspect, with a large size diameter, up to 10 um, a complex morphology, with dendritic spines invaginated in the boutons, and a high synaptic vesicles density [9-12].

Biochemistry of Granule Cells and Mossy Fibers During Development

The MF ending nerves are enriched in zinc [13,14]. Zinc is first detected in the granular layer by day PN 18 and in the region of MF terminals, the *stratum lucidum*, between days PN 18 and 22, in rat [15]. The apparition of zinc in the MF ending nerves is concomitant to the development of the MFs.

In the adult brain, γ-aminobutyric acid (GABA) is the main inhibitory neurotransmitter and the neurotransmitter of interneurons [16,17]. During the first week postnatal, granule cells express a GABAergic phenotype; granule cells are immunoreactive for GABA and glutamate decarboxylase (GAD) 67 [18,19]. GAD is the biosynthetic enzyme for GABA [20,21]. The GABAergic phenotype of granule cells is downregulated, concomitantly to the development of GABAergic inhibition in the CA3 region, mediated by interneurons, and the development of the glutamatergic phenotype of granule cells and MFs [22].

The expression of a GABAergic phenotype by an excitatory glutamatergic population of nerve cells raises the question of its significance and physiological role during development.

GABA a Transient Excitatory Transmitter During Development

In the developing nervous system, it is well established that GABA could function transiently as an excitatory transmitter [23-28] and elicit trophic activities, particularly promoting synaptogenesis [29-32].

During the first week postnatal, contrary to the adult, GABA exerts a depolarizing activity on CA3 hippocampal neurons [22,25]. The depolarization of CA3 hippocampal neurons induced by GABA during the first week of development enables N-methyl-D-aspartate receptors to activate CA3 hippocampal neurons [33].

The excitatory effect of GABA during development becomes inhibitory as the neurons mature. From the second week postnatal, GABA exerts an inhibitory hyperpolarizing activity on CA3 pyramidal cells [34], at a time when pyramidal cells mature and acquire their adult features [4,11]. GABA exerting a depolarizing activity onto CA3 pyramidal cells would originate from hilar and CA3 interneurons of the hippocampus.

In addition, during the postnatal period, granule cells express a GABAergic phenotype; granule cells are immunoreactive for GABA and glutamate decarboxylase (GAD) 67 [18,19]. The GABAergic phenotype of granule cells is downregulated, concomitantly to the establishment of GABAergic inhibition in CA3, mediated by interneurons or disynaptic inhibition, and the development of the MF glutamatergic phenotype [22]. This suggests that MF-GABAergic transmission accompanies the morphological maturation of pyramidal cells, possibly until the completion of the development of dendrites and spines, which happens at approximately the same time [12].

In the mature nervous system, GABA is the main inhibitory neurotransmitter and the neurotransmitter of interneurons system [16,17]. The activity of the fast acting neurotransmitter GABA is mediated through its interaction with the GABA(A) receptors (GABA(A)-Rs) [35]. The GABA(A)-R is coupled to the opening of chloride ion (Cl^-) channels. Upon interaction of GABA with GABA(A)-Rs, the opening of Cl^- channels leads to an influx of Cl^- inside the cells and hyperpolarization of the nerve cells' membrane potential [35]. This underlies the inhibitory activity of GABA on nerve cells. It is proposed that a transient reversal of the distribution of Cl^- in nerve cells underlies the switch of GABA activity from hyperpolarizing to depolarizing, during development [36-38].

GABA originating from granule cells could contribute to the depolarization of the CA3 pyramidal cells by adding to the GABAergic input of the hilar and CA3 interneurons. After completion of development, the expression of the GABAergic phenotype by the granule cells is downregulated, establishing the adult interneuron-mediated disynaptic inhibition onto CA3 pyramidal cells.

The depolarizing activity of GABA onto CA3 pyramidal cells would exert a trophic effect on these cells during development [39-41]. The transient expression of GABAergic phenotype by granule cells may contribute to the trophic effect of GABA during development and support the glutamate-GABA synergism on developing postsynaptic cells. In the adult brain, GABA is colocalized with glutamate in MF terminals [35]. The expression of a GABAergic phenotype in the adult MFs may be reminiscent of the development.

AFFERENT FIBERS

Major afferent fibers to the hippocampus reach their targets after the presumptive fields of CA3 and CA1 are in place. Afferent fibers from the septum arrive in the mouse hippocampus at day E 17.5 and afferent fibers from the entorhinal cortex reach the DG at day E 19.5 [2].

CONCLUSION

Contrary to other neuronal cell populations, hippocampal dentate granule cells develop mainly postnatally. Hence, granule cells originating at different stages coexist in the hippocampus. The development of both the DG and CA shows a striking coordination and gradual specification, with the CA region specified early during the embryonic development and the DG mostly during the first two weeks postnatal.

The developing hippocampus during the prenatal period is divided into two presumptive fields that prefigure the mature CA1 and CA3 fields. These two regions were originally termed presumptive CA1 and CA3 (Pca1 and Pca3) and can be distinguished in the mouse several days before birth by a complementary pattern of gene expression, for SCIP and kainate receptor gene, a pattern conserved throughout adulthood [43,44]. This shows that certain genes are expressed in specific hippocampal subfields during development and their expression is preserved through adulthood [43,44].

During the maturation process, granule cells express transiently a GABAergic phenotype. This GABAergic phenotype, eliciting a depolarizing activity onto CA3 pyramidal cells, contributes to the trophic effect of GABA during development, particularly on the MF synaptogenesis and maturation of CA3 pyramidal cells. Additional investigations are needed to establish whether glutamate and GABA are released from the same MF terminals and how the proportion of release of both amino acids varies during development. This phenotypic plasticity of granule cells may not only contribute to developmental functions, but also in protective effects during seizures in the young.

Contrary to a long-held belief that the development of the mammalian nervous system occurs primarily prenatally, with most nerve cells born before birth, neurogenesis occurs throughout adulthood in discrete regions of the brain, including in humans, and neural stem cells reside in the adult central nervous system suggesting that the development of the brain may never end [45-48].

REFERENCES

[1] Angevine JB. (1965) Time of neuron origin in the hippocampal region; an autoradiographic study in the mouse. *Exp Neurol. 13*, 1-70.

[2] Super H, Soriano E. (1994) The organization of the embryonic and early postnatal murine hippocampus. II. Development of entorhinal, commissural, and septal connections studied with the lipophilic tracer DiI. *J Comp Neurol. 344*, 101-20.

[3] Stanfield BB, Cowan WM. (1984) An EM autoradiographic study of the hypothalamo-hippocampal projection. *Brain Res. 309*, 299-307.

[4] Zimmer J. (1978) Development of the hippocampus and fascia dentata: morphological and histochemical aspects. *Prog Brain Res. 48*, 171-90.

[5] Woodhams PL, Webb M, Atkinson DJ, Seeley PJ. (1989) A monoclonal antibody, Py, distinguishes different classes of hippocampal neurons. *J Neurosci. 9*, 2170-81.

[6] Lai C, Gore M, Lemke G. (1994) Structure, expression, and activity of Tyro 3, a neural adhesion-related receptor tyrosine kinase. *Oncogene. 9*, 2567-78.

[7] Grove EA, Tole S. (1999) Patterning events and specification signals in the developing hippocampus. *Cereb Cortex. 9*, 551-61.

[8] Tole S, Christian C, Grove EA. (1997) Early specification and autonomous development of cortical fields in the mouse hippocampus. *Development. 124*, 4959-70.

[9] Gaarskjaer FB. (1986) The organization and development of the hippocampal mossy fiber system. *Brain Res. 396*, 335-57.

[10] Altman J, Bayer SA. (1990) Migration and distribution of two populations of hippocampal granule cell precursors during the perinatal and postnatal periods. *J Comp Neurol. 301*, 365-81.

[11] Bayer SA. (1980) Development of the hippocampal region in the rat. II. Morphogenesis during embryonic and early postnatal life. *J Comp Neurol. 190*, 115-34.

[12] Amaral DG, Dent JA. (1981) Development of the mossy fibers of the dentate gyrus: I. A light and electron microscopic study of the mossy fibers and their expansions. *J Comp Neurol. 195*, 51-86.

[13] McLardy T. (1962) Zinc enzymes and the hippocampal mossy fibre system. *Nature. 194*, 300-2.

[14] Haug FMS. (1967) Electron microscopical localization of the zinc in hippocampal mossy fiber synapses by a modified sulfide silver procedure. *Histochimie. 8*, 355-68.

[15] Crawford Il, Connor JD. (1972) Zinc in maturing rat brain: hippocampal concentration and localization. *J. Neurochem. 19*, 1451-8.

[16] Ribak CE, Seress L. (1983) Five types of basket cell in the hippocampal dentate gyrus: a combined Golgi and electron microscopic study. *J Neurocytol. 12*, 577-97.

[17] Seress L, Ribak CE. (1983) GABAergic cells in the dentate gyrus appear to be local circuit and projection neurons. *Exp Brain Res. 50*, 173-82.

[18] Dupuy ST, Houser CR. (1996) Prominent expression of two forms of glutamate decarboxylase in the embryonic and early postnatal rat hippocampal formation. *J Neurosci. 16*, 6919-32.

[19] Dupuy ST, Houser CR. (1997) Developmental changes in GABA neurons of the rat dentate gyrus: an in situ hybridization and birthdating study. J Comp Neurol. 389, 402-18.

[20] Roberts E, Frankel S. (1950) Aminobutyric acid in brain: its formation from glutamic acid. *J Biol Chem. 187*, 55-63.

[21] Erlander MG, Tillakaratne NJ, Feldblum S, Patel N, Tobin AJ. (1991) Two genes encode distinct glutamate decarboxylases. *Neuron. 7*, 91-100.

[22] Hennou S, Khalilov I, Diabira D, Ben-Ari Y, Gozlan H. (2002) Early sequential formation of functional GABA(A) and glutamatergic synapses on CA1 interneurons of the rat foetal hippocampus. *Eur J Neurosci. 16*, 197-208.

[23] Ben-Ari Y, Cherubini E, Corradetti R, Gaiarsa JL. (1989) Giant synaptic potentials in immature rat CA3 hippocampal neurones. *J Physiol. 416*, 303-25.

[24] LoTurco JJ, Owens DF, Heath MJ, Davis MB, Kriegstein AR. (1995) GABA and glutamate depolarize cortical progenitor cells and inhibit DNA synthesis. *Neuron. 15*, 1287-98.

[25] Cherubini E, Rovira C, Gaiarsa JL, Corradetti R, Ben Ari Y. (1990) GABA mediated excitation in immature rat CA3 hippocampal neurons. *Int J Dev Neurosci. 8*, 481-90.

[26] Owens DF, Boyce LH, Davis MB, Kriegstein AR. (1996) Excitatory GABA responses in embryonic and neonatal cortical slices demonstrated by gramicidin perforated-patch recordings and calcium imaging. *J Neurosci. 16*, 6414-23.

[27] Khalilov I, Dzhala V, Ben-Ari Y, Khazipov R. (1999) Dual role of GABA in the neonatal rat hippocampus. *Dev Neurosci. 21*, 310-9.

[28] Leinekugel X, Khalilov I, McLean H, Caillard O, Gaiarsa JL, Ben-Ari Y, Khazipov R. (1999) GABA is the principal fast-acting excitatory transmitter in the neonatal brain. *Adv Neurol. 79*, 189-201.

[29] Madtes P Jr, Redburn DA. (1983) GABA as a trophic factor during development. *Life Sci. 33*, 979-84.

[30] Spoerri PE. (1988) Neurotrophic effects of GABA in cultures of embryonic chick brain and retina. *Synapse. 2*, 11-22.

[31] Barbin G, Pollard H, Gaiarsa JL, Ben-Ari Y. (1993) Involvement of GABAA receptors in the outgrowth of cultured hippocampal neurons. *Neurosci Lett. 152*, 150-4.

[32] Zafra F, Castren E, Thoenen H, Lindholm D. (1991) Interplay between glutamate and gamma-aminobutyric acid transmitter systems in the physiological regulation of brain-derived neurotrophic factor and nerve growth factor synthesis in hippocampal neurons. *Proc Natl Acad Sci U S A. 88*, 10037-41.

[33] Leinekugel X, Medina I, Khalilov I, Ben-Ari Y, Khazipov R. (1997) Ca2+ oscillations mediated by the synergistic excitatory actions of GABA(A) and NMDA receptors in the neonatal hippocampus. *Neuron. 18*, 243-55.

[34] Gaiarsa JL, McLean H, Congar P, Leinekugel X, Khazipov R, Tseeb V, Ben-Ari Y. (1995) Postnatal maturation of gamma-aminobutyric acidA and B-mediated inhibition in the CA3 hippocampal region of the rat. *J Neurobiol. 26*, 339-49.

[35] Sivilotti L, Nistri A. (1991) GABA receptor mechanisms in the central nervous system. *Progress in Neurobiology. 36*, 35-92.

[36] Cherubini E, Gaiarsa JL, Ben-Ari Y. (1991) GABA: an excitatory transmitter in early postnatal life. *Trends Neurosci. 14*, 515-9.

[37] Michelson HB, Wong RK. (1991) Excitatory synaptic responses mediated by GABAA receptors in the hippocampus. *Science. 253*, 1420-3.

[38] Ben-Ari Y. (2002) Excitatory actions of gaba during development: the nature of the nurture. *Nat Rev Neurosci. 3*, 728-39.

[39] Ben-Ari Y, Tseeb V, Raggozzino D, Khazipov R, Gaiarsa JL. (1994) Gamma-Aminobutyric acid (GABA): a fast excitatory transmitter which may regulate the development of hippocampal neurones in early postnatal life. *Prog Brain Res. 102*, 261-73.

[40] Ben-Ari Y, Khazipov R, Leinekugel X, Caillard O, Gaiarsa JL. (1997) GABAA, NMDA and AMPA receptors: a developmentally regulated 'menage a trois'. *Trends Neurosci. 20*, 523-9.

[41] Ben-Ari Y. (2001) Developing networks play a similar melody. *Trends Neurosci. 24*, 353-60.

[42] Sandler R, Smith AD. (1991) Coexistence of GABA and glutamate in mossy fiber terminals of the primate hippocampus: an ultrastructural study. *J Comp Neurol. 303*, 177-92.

[43] Wisden W, Seeburg PH. (1993) A complex mosaic of high-affinity kainate receptors in rat brain. *J Neurosci. 13*, 3582-98.

[44] Lemke G, Kuhn R, Monuki ES, Weinmaster G. (1991) Expression and activity of the transcription factor SCIP during glial differentiation and myelination. *Ann N Y Acad Sci. 633*, 189-95.

[45] Gage FH. (2000) Mammalian neural stem cells. *Science. 287*, 1433-8.

[46] Gross CG. (2000) Neurogenesis in the adult brain: death of a dogma. *Nat Rev Neurosci. 1*, 67-73.

[47] Kaplan MS. (2001) Environment complexity stimulates visual cortex neurogenesis: death of a dogma and a research career. *Trends Neurosci. 24*, 617-20.

[48] Taupin P, Gage FH. (2002) Adult neurogenesis and neural stem cells of the central nervous system in mammals. *J Neurosci Res. 69*, 745-9.

Chapter IX

Adult Neurogenesis and Neural Stem Cells

Abstract

Contrary to a long-held dogma, neurogenesis, the generation of new neuronal cells, occurs throughout adulthood in mammals. Neurogenesis occurs primarily in two discrete regions of the adult brain, the subventricular zone (SVZ) lining the ventricles and dentate gyrus (DG) of the hippocampus, in various species including humans. It is postulated that newly generated neuronal cells originate from stem cells in the adult brain. Neural stem cells (NSCs) are the self-renewing multipotent cells that generate the main phenotypes of the nervous system. A glial origin for newly generated neuronal cells in the SVZ and DG has been proposed. In the adult brain, neurogenesis may recapitulate a developmental process. Neural progenitor and stem cells have also been isolated and characterized *in vitro*, from various regions of the adult central nervous system (CNS) and species, including human *post mortem* tissues. Adult neurogenesis is modulated by a broad range of environmental, and physio- and pathological conditions, as well as trophic factors/cytokines and drugs. Newly generated neuronal cells in the adult brain may be involved in learning and memory, depression, regenerative attempts and plasticity. The confirmation that neurogenesis occurs in the adult brain and NSCs reside in the adult CNS suggests that the development of the brain may never end and the CNS may be amenable to repair.

Introduction

Multipotent stem cells are self-renewing cells that generate the main cell types of the tissue in which they reside. Multipotent stem cells are present in fetal and adult tissues. In the fetus, they contribute to development of the tissues and in the adult to homeostasis of the tissues and regeneration after injuries [1]. In the mammalian CNS, most nerve cells are born during the prenatal phase of development, with the exception of the granule cells of the DG of the hippocampus, which are mostly born during the first two weeks postnatal [2-4]. It was believed that the adult brain lacks the capacity to generate new nerve cells, dogma known as "no new neuron dogma". An underlying reason for this belief was that the adult brain was devoid of stem cells, which took support from the limited capacity of the adult CNS to recover from injuries [5].

In the early 60s, Altman and Altman and Das published several seminal studies reporting the generation of new neuronal cells in discrete areas of the adult brain, the SVZ and DG, in rodents [6-9]. These studies were substantiated in the 70s and early 80s [10,11]. Adult neurogenesis was thought to be limited to lower mammals and songbirds [12,13], as it was not reported in primates [14]. In the 80s and 90s, with the advent of new methods for labeling dividing cells, like bromodeoxyurine (5-bromo-2'-deoxyuridine, BrdU) labeling, retroviral labeling and confocal microscopy, investigators confirmed that neurogenesis occurs in discrete areas of the mammalian brain throughout adulthood in various species, including primates [15-18]. BrdU is a thymidine analog used for birthdating and monitoring cell proliferation [19,20]. Retroviruses infect only dividing cells and allow the detection of newly generated cells' origin, lineage and fate, as well as tracking cell migration and physiological studies [21]. It is postulated that newly generated neuronal cells originate from stem cells in the adult brain. The existence of NSCs in the adult mammalian brain has tremendous consequences for our understanding of development and functioning of the CNS, as well as for therapy. The development of the CNS may never end and the CNS may be amenable to repair.

Neurogenesis in the Adult Brain

Neurogenesis occurs primarily in two regions of the forebrain in adult mammals, the SVZ and DG, in various species, including humans [15-18]. The SVZ is a layer of cells along the ventricle. It is reminiscent of the embryonic ventricular zone, site of origin of neural progenitor and stem cells during development. In the anterior part of the SVZ, newly generated neuronal cells migrate to the olfactory bulb (OB), through the rostro-migratory stream (RMS), in rodents [22-25] and in primates, non-human and human [26-29]. In the OB, they differentiate into functional interneurons, granule and periglomerular neurons. Newly generated neuronal cells in the SVZ aggregate to form a network of chains of neuroblasts [30]. These neuroblast chains migrate tangentially through the SVZ and coalesce anteriorly to form the RMS (figure 1) [31]. In humans, the RMS is organized, differently than in other species, around a lateral ventricular extension reaching the OB [29,32]. In rodents (mice), a SVZ progenitor cell requires at least 15 days to be generated, migrate 3-5 mm and differentiate into new olfactory interneurons. These cells migrate at an average rate of 30 μm/hr [24]. In monkeys (macaque), a SVZ progenitor cell requires at least 75 to 97 days to be generated, migrate 20 mm and differentiate into new olfactory interneurons, a process slower than in rodents [26].

In the DG, newly generated neuronal cells in the subgranular zone (SGZ) migrate to the granule cell layer, where they differentiate into neuronal cells, extend axonal projections to the *Cornu Ammonis* (CA) region CA3 and establish functional connections, in rodents [33-36] and primates, non-human and human (figure 2) [37-39]. The SGZ is a layer beneath the granular layer of the DG. In rodents (rat), immature granule cells extend axons into CA3 as rapidly as 4-10 days after mitosis [40], whereas the maturation of newborn cells, from the proliferation of newly generated cells in the SGZ to the migration and differentiation into neuronal cells of the granule cell layer, takes approximately 4 weeks [33].

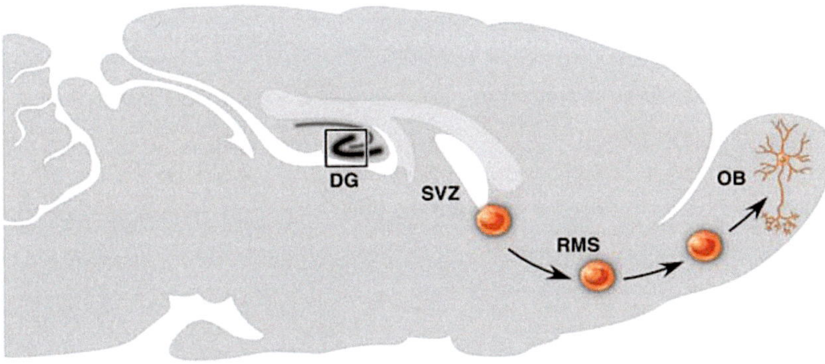

Figure 1. Neurogenesis in the adult subventricular zone. Neurogenesis occurs primarily in two regions of the adult mammalian brain, the subventricular zone (SVZ) and dentate gyrus (DG), in various species, including humans. The SVZ is a layer of cells along the ventricle. In the anterior part of the SVZ, newborn neuronal cells migrate to the olfactory bulb (OB), through the rostro-migratory stream (RMS). In the OB, they differentiate into interneurons, granule and periglomerular neurons. In human, the RMS is organized, differently than in other species, around a lateral ventricular extension reaching the OB.

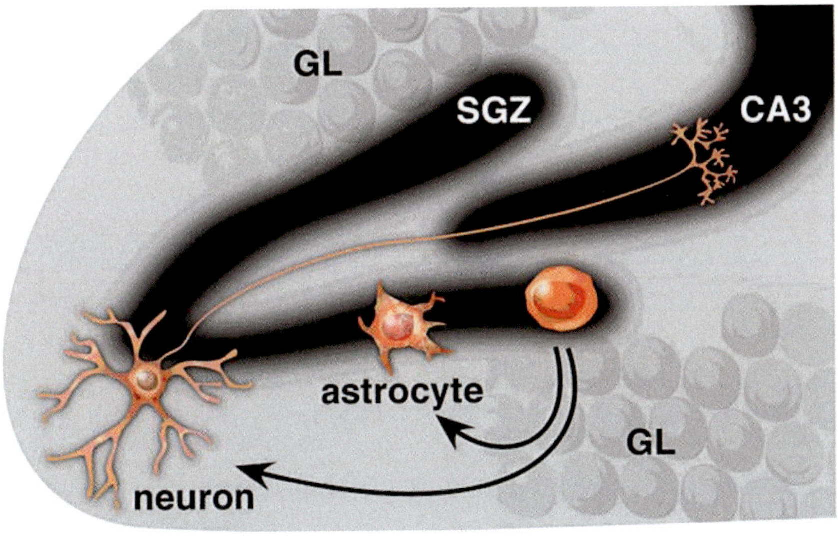

Figure 2. Neurogenesis in the adult dentate gyrus. The hippocampus is divided in two regions, the dentate gyrus and *Cornu Ammonis*. In the dentate gyrus (DG), newborn neuronal cells in the subgranular zone (SGZ) migrate to the granule layer (GL), where they differentiate into neuronal cells and astrocytes. The SGZ is a layer beneath the granular layer of the DG. The GL is the principal cell layer of the DG. Newly generated neuronal cells in the GL extend axonal projections to the *Cornu Ammonis* region CA3.

Of these two regions, the SVZ harbors the largest pool of dividing neural progenitor cells [23,31,33]. Cell death is a normally occurring process in the adult brain and particularly for newly generated cells in the neurogenic zones [41,42]. As many as 9,000 new neuronal cells are generated per day in the rodent DG, contributing to about 3.3% per month or about 0.1% per day of the granule cell population [42,43], whereas in adult macaque monkey, it is estimated that at least 0.004% of the neuronal population in the granule cell layer are new neurons generated per day [38]. The rate of neurogenesis in the human DG was also reported to be low [39]. The relative rate of neurogenesis is estimated to be approximately 10 times lower in adult macaque monkeys than that reported in the adult rodent DG [38].

The reasons for the apparent decline of adult neurogenesis in primates are unclear. The decline of adult neurogenesis during vertebrate evolution could be an adaptive strategy to maintain stable neuronal populations throughout life [14]. This hypothesis is consistent with the restriction of adult neurogenesis in the mammalian brain to phylogenetically older structures, like the OB and hippocampus, and its absence in the more recently evolved neocortex [44,45]. However, as most studies use BrdU to quantify neurogenesis, it remains difficult to make comparisons between species, as nothing is known about the ability of BrdU to cross the blood-brain barrier and be available for uptake by dividing cells between different species [20]. These data must therefore be taken cautiously.

Neurogenesis may also occur in other areas of the adult brain -albeit at lower level- in certain species, like the CA1 area [46], the neocortex [47,48], the striatum [49], the amygdala [50], the substantia nigra [51]. However some of these data have been the sources of debates and controversies and remain to be further confirmed [20,45,52-54].

Altogether neurogenesis occurs in the adult mammalian brain. Newborn granule cells in the DG survive for extended period of time, at least 2 years in humans [39]. This suggests that neuronal cells born during adulthood that become integrated into circuits and survive to maturity are very stable. They may permanently replace granule cells born during development.

Origin of Newly Generated Neuronal Cells in the Adult Brain

Based on ultrastructure, cell cycle analysis, [3H]-thymidine autoradiography, immunohistochemical studies, particularly BrdU-labeling, retroviral labeling and studies in transgenic mice, investigators have aimed at identifying the origin of newly generated neuronal cells in the adult mammalian brain. Two theories have been proposed. One theory contends that newly generated neuronal cells originate from astrocyte-like cells, expressing the intermediate filaments glial fibrillary acidic protein (GFAP) and nestin, in the SVZ and hippocampus [55-61]. GFAP is an intermediate filament marker of mature glial cells [62]. Nestin is an intermediate filament considered as marker of neuroepithelial and CNS stem cells [63,64]. The second theory contends that newly generated neuronal cells originate from a population of ependymal cells in the SVZ that express nestin [65]. The ependyma and subependyma originate from the embryonic forebrain germinal zones.

On the one hand, the finding that a population of astrocyte-like cells is at the origin of newly generated neuronal cells in the adult brain is surprising, as astrocytes are differentiated cells belonging to the glial lineage. On the other hand, the ependymal origin of newly generated neuronal cells in the SVZ is not supported by other studies [66,67]. Though more recent reports further support a glial origin for newly generated neuronal cells in the adult brain [68-70], their origin remains to be unequivocally determined [18].

A Developmental Process

In the mature nervous system, γ-aminobutyric acid (GABA) is an inhibitory neurotransmitter and the main neurotransmitter of interneurons [71,72]. In birds, GABAergic neurons participate in the brain's response to auditory stimulation [73].

In mammals, during the development of the nervous system, GABAergic synapses are formed prior to glutamatergic ones [74] and GABA acts as an excitatory neurotransmitter [75]. Granule cells of the hippocampal DG develop mostly during the first two weeks postnatal [2,3]. During the first postnatal week, contrary to the mature hippocampus, GABA exerts a depolarizing effect on CA3 hippocampal neurons [76,77]. The depolarizing activity of GABA onto CA3 pyramidal cells would regulate synaptic integration and survival of newly generated neuronal cells, and exert a trophic activity on these cells during development [78-81]. The depolarizing activity of GABA would originate from an increased chloride levels in immature neuronal cells [82].

In the adult brain, newly generated neuronal cells in the DG receive GABAergic innervations soon after their migration is completed [83]. The GABAergic synaptic input on neural precursor cells of the SVZ and DG has a depolarizing activity on these cells, providing an excitatory input on newborn neuronal cells of the adult brain [84- 86]. The origin and mechanism of the GABA innervation on newly generated neuronal cells of the adult brain remain to be determined. It would result from an increased chloride levels in immature neuronal cells, as during development [82]. In the adult brain, GABAergic depolarization of newly generated neural progenitor cells in the adult brain triggers the expression of NeuroD; a transcription factor required for the maturation of hippocampal dentate granule cells [86].

The depolarizing activity of GABA in the adult brain would exert a trophic activity and regulate synaptic integration of neural precursor cells, as during development [87,88]. In support to this contention, in the SVZ and RMS, GABA released by astrocyte-like cells controls the proliferation and migration of neuronal precursors [89,90]. Adult neurogenesis may reproduce processes similar as during development, to integrate newborn neuronal cells in the hippocampal network [91].

Neural Progenitor and Stem Cells of the Adult Brain

It is postulated that newly generated neuronal cells originate from residual stem cells in the adult brain [15,18]. Stem cells are defined as cells with the capacity to proliferate, self-renew over an extended period of time, generate of a large number of differentiated progeny and regenerate the tissue following injury. Progenitor cells are, as most broadly defined, any cells that do not fulfill all of the criteria defining stem cells [1]. Neural stem cells (NSCs) are the self-renewing multipotent cells that generate, through a transient amplifying population of cells, i.e., neural progenitor cells, the main phenotypes of the nervous system, neurons, astrocytes and oligodendrocytes (figure 3).

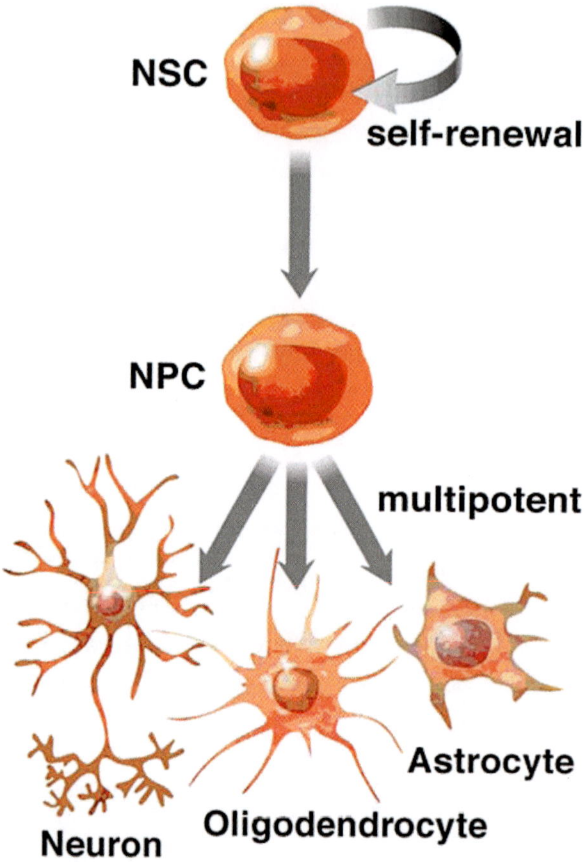

Figure 3. Neural progenitor and stem cells. Neural stem cells (NSCs) are the self-renewing multipotent cells that generate, through a transient amplifying population of cells, i.e., neural progenitor cells (NPCs), the main phenotypes of the nervous system, neurons, astrocytes and oligodendrocytes. It is postulated that newborn neuronal cells originate from residual stem cells in the adult brain.

In 1992, Reynolds and Weiss were the first to isolate and characterize *in vitro*, from the adult brain tissue, neural progenitor and stem cells expressing the neuroepithelial and CNS stem cell marker nestin. The neural progenitor and stem cells were isolated from the striatal area, including the SVZ [92]. Since then self-renewing multipotent neural progenitor and stem cells have been isolated and characterized *in vitro*, from various areas of the CNS, like the hippocampus and spinal cord, and species, including from human *post mortem* tissues [53,93-100]. These results show that neural progenitor and stem cells isolated and cultured *in vitro* are heterogeneous populations of cells and that neural progenitor and stem cells reside throughout the adult CNS [101,102].

In fact, NSCs are still elusive cells in the adult CNS and remain to be unequivocally identified and characterized. The isolation and characterization of neural progenitor and stem cells from the adult human brain provide a source of tissue for cellular therapy.

MODULATION AND PHYSIOPATHOLOGY

Neurogenesis in the DG and SVZ is modulated by a broad range of environmental, and physio- and pathological conditions, as well as trophic factors/cytokines and drugs [103]. Most of these investigations were performed using BrdU-labeling paradigm. Neurogenesis decreases with age and stress [104,105]. Learning and memory tasks, environmental enrichment and voluntary exercises enhance neurogenesis [43,106,107]. Neurogenesis is stimulated in the DG and SVZ, in the diseased brain and after CNS injuries, like in Alzheimer's and Huntington's diseases, epilepsia, cerebral strokes and ischemia, and traumatic brain injuries [108-112] (table 1). The confirmation and evidence, that neurogenesis occurs and is modulated in the DG and SVZ, raise the question of the function of newborn neuronal cells in the adult brain.

Reports show that newly generated neuronal cells in the hippocampus are involved in learning and memory, and depression [113-115]. The function of newborn neuronal cells in learning and memory has been challenged by other studies. On the one hand, enhanced hippocampal neurogenesis has been observed without improvement of learning and memory performances, and learning enhances the survival of new neurons beyond the time required for memory performance [116,117]. On the other hand, nonspecific effects of treatments aiming at inhibiting adult neurogenesis have yet to be ruled out [118]. There are also controversies and debates over the involvement of adult neurogenesis in the etiology depression. Among them, the hippocampus may not be primarily involved in depressive episodes, as other areas of the brain may play a critical role in depression. There are also questions over the validity of animal models of depression, as representative of the human disorder [119-121].

New neuronal cells are generated at the sites of degeneration where they replace some of the degenerated nerve cells, after experimental strokes [122,123]. New neuronal cells at the sites of degeneration originate from the SVZ; they migrate to the sites of degeneration partially through the RMS. An estimated 0.2% of the degenerated nerve cells are replaced in the striatum after middle cerebral artery occlusion, a model of focal ischemia [122,123]. This suggests that adult neurogenesis may be involved in attempts to regenerate the brain tissue in the diseased and injured CNS.

There are pitfalls and limitations over the use of BrdU labeling to study neurogenesis [20]. Various physio- and pathological conditions are known to affect the permeability of the blood-brain barrier [124,125]. Abortive cell cycle reentry, as a prelude to apoptosis, and gene duplication without cell proliferation have been reported to occur in the brain in various models of CNS diseases and injuries [126-130]. BrdU is also known to have toxic and mutagenic effects [131-133]. All of which may affect the validity of BrdU-labeling for studying neurogenesis [20]. Caution must be taken when using standard protocols, like BrdU-labeling, for studying neurogenesis. Further investigations are required to confirm the involvement of adult neurogenesis in various physio- and pathological conditions.

Table 1. Modulation of neurogenesis in the adult brain

Stimuli	Area	Modulation	Reference #
Environment			
Environmental enrichment	DG	increase	43, 144
Learning task	DG	increase	106
Physical activity	DG	increase	107, 145
Alcohol consumption	DG	decrease	146-148
Dietary supplement	DG	increase	149, 150
Maternal deprivation	DG	decrease	151
Social isolation	DG	decrease	152
Stress	DG	decrease	153
Physiological conditions			
Age	DG, SVZ, OB	decrease	154-156
Estrous cycle	DG, SVZ	increase during proestrus	157, 158
Alzheimer's disease			
Autopsy	DG	increase	112
PSEN1 mutant (*)	DG, SVZ	decrease	159
APP mutant/Swedish (*)	DG, SVZ	increase	160
Huntington's disease	DG	increase	111
Epilepsy			
Pilocarpine-induced seizures	DG	increase	108, 161
Kainic acid-induced seizures	DG	increase	161-163
Kindling stimulation	DG	increase	163

Neurogenesis occurs throughout adulthood primarily in two regions of the brain, the dentate gyrus (DG) and subventricular zone (SVZ). Newly generated neuronal cells in the SVZ migrate to the olfactory bulb (OB), through the rostro-migratory stream. Neurogenesis in the DG and SVZ is modulated by a broad range of environmental, and physio- and pathlogical conditions. (*) Adult neurogenesis has been characterized in animal models of Alzheimer's disease, like knock-out mice for the gene presenilin 1 (PSEN1) and transgenic mice expressing the Swedish and Indiana amyloid precursor protein (APP) mutations, a mutant form of human APP.

In all, neurogenesis may be involved in a broad range of physio- and pathological conditions. However, the contribution of newborn neuronal cells to these events must be confirmed and sorted out from potential artifacts. It is proposed that adult neurogenesis may be involved in CNS plasticity. Neuroplasticity is the ability of the CNS to reorganize neural pathways based on new experiences [134]. Neurogenesis in the adult brain would contribute to CNS plasticity in reorganizing neural pathways as a result of new experiences [135]. The contribution of adult neurogenesis to the other components of CNS plasticity, like axonal sprouting, reorganization of the contra-lateral hemisphere, to the functioning and physiopathology of the CNS remains to be determined.

CELLULAR THERAPY

The confirmation that neurogenesis occurs in the adult brain and NSCs reside in the adult CNS suggests that the adult mammalian CNS may be amenable to repair. Cell therapeutic intervention may involve the stimulation and transplantation of neural progenitor and stem cells of the adult CNS.

In vitro isolation and characterization of neural progenitor and stem cells reveals that those cells may reside throughout the adult CNS. Hence, the stimulation of endogenous neural progenitor and stem cells locally would represent a strategy to promote regeneration in the diseased brain and after CNS injuries. Alternatively, new neuronal cells are generated at sites of degeneration after CNS injuries, like strokes [122,123]. These cells originate from the SVZ and migrate partially through the RMS to the sites of degeneration. Strategies to promote regeneration and repair may focus on stimulating SVZ neurogenesis.

Neural progenitor and stem cells can be isolated from the adult brain, including from human biopsies and *post mortem* tissues [95,96], providing valuable sources of tissue for cellular therapy. In support of this contention, fetal-derived neural progenitor and stem cells have been grafted in various animals model of CNS diseases and injuries, like Parkinson's disease and spinal cord injuries, and shown to improve functional recovery [136-141]. In these studies, the release of trophic factors by the grafted neural progenitor and stem cells, their interaction with the injured brain and the immune system are believed to play major roles in the recovery process [136,138-140]. In a study where human fetal neural progenitor and stem cells were injected after spinal cord injury in mice, the improvements in walking disappeared following treatment with diphtheria toxin, which kills only human cells -not mouse cells- [141]. This suggests that the grafted cells themselves are responsible for recovery.

These studies provide the proof-of-principle of the potential of neural progenitor and stem cells for therapy and reveal that administration of stem cells might contribute directly to repair damage in the injured CNS [141]. Adult-derived neural progenitor and stem cells may also provide the opportunity to perform autologous transplantation, in which neural progenitor and stem cells isolated from an undamaged area would be cultured *in vitro* and grafted to the patient himself. However, risk associated with invasive surgical procedure that would probably involves the destruction of healthy brain tissue, limits the clinical application of such strategy [142-143].

CONCLUSION

The confirmation that neurogenesis occurs in the adult brain and that NSCs reside in the adult CNS has tremendous implications for our understanding of the development and functioning of the nervous system, as well as for cellular therapy. Over the past decade, significant progress has been made in this field of research. However, fundamental issues remain to be resolved. Among them, why does neurogenesis occur primarily in discrete regions of the adult brain? What is the origin of newly generated neuronal cells in the adult brain? What are the mechanisms underlying adult neurogenesis *in vitro* and *in vivo*? What are the markers defining neural stem versus progenitor cells? Can homogenous populations of neural progenitor or stem cells be maintained in culture? What is the function(s) of newly generated neuronal cells in the adult brain? How to bring adult NSCs to therapy? Adult NSCs offer new and promising opportunities to treat a broad range of diseases and injuries of the nervous system, like Alzheimer's and Parkinson's diseases. The answer to these questions is a prerequisite to bring adult NSCs to therapy.

Acknowledgments

Chapter 9, figures 1, 2 and 3, are reprinted, with permission, from from *J Neurosci Res*, Vol 69, Taupin P, Gage FH, Adult neurogenesis and neural stem cells of the central nervous system in mammals, Pages 745-9, Copyright (2002), Wiley-Liss, Inc., a subsidiary of John Wiley & Sons, Inc.

References

[1] Potten CS, Loeffler M. (1990) Stem cells: attributes, cycles, spirals, pitfalls and uncertainties. Lessons for and from the crypt. *Development. 110*, 1001-20.

[2] Bayer SA. (1980) Development of the hippocampal region in the rat. II. Morphogenesis during embryonic and early postnatal life. *J Comp Neurol. 190*, 115-34.

[3] Gaarskjaer FB. (1986) The organization and development of the hippocampal mossy fiber system. *Brain Research Reviews. 11*, 335-57.

[4] Kandel ER, Schwartz JH, Jessell TM. *Principles of Neural Science*. Publisher: McGraw-Hill Medical; 4 edition (January 5, 2000).

[5] Santiago Ramon y Cajal. *Degeneration and Regeneration of the Nervous System*. New York: Hafner (1928).

[6] Altman J. (1962) Are new neurons formed in the brains of adult mammals? *Science.135*, 1127-8.

[7] Altman J. (1963) Autoradiographic investigation of cell proliferation in the brains of rats and cats. *Anat Rec. 145*, 573-91.

[8] Altman J, Das GD. (1965) Autoradiographic and histological evidence of postnatal hippocampal neurogenesis in rats. *J Comp Neurol. 124*, 319-36.

[9] Altman J. (1969) Autoradiographic and histological studies of postnatal neurogenesis. IV. Cell proliferation and migration in the anterior forebrain, with special reference to persisting neurogenesis in the olfactory bulb. *J Comp Neurol. 137*, 433-58.

[10] Kaplan MS, Hinds JW. (1977) Neurogenesis in the adult rat: electron microscopic analysis of light radioautographs. *Science. 197*, 1092-4.

[11] Bayer SA, Yackel JW, Puri PS. (1982) Neurons in the rat dentate gyrus granular layer substantially increase during juvenile and adult life. *Science. 216*, 890-2.

[12] Goldman SA, Nottebohm F. (1983) Neuronal production, migration, and differentiation in a vocal control nucleus of the adult female canary brain. *Proc Natl Acad Sci U S A. 80*, 2390-4.

[13] Nottebohm F. (2004) The road we travelled: discovery, choreography, and significance of brain replaceable neurons. *Ann N Y Acad Sci. 1016*, 628-58.

[14] Rakic P. (1985) Limits of neurogenesis in primates. *Science. 227*, 1054-6.

[15] Gage FH. (2000) Mammalian neural stem cells. *Science. 287*, 1433-8.

[16] Gross CG. (2000) Neurogenesis in the adult brain: death of a dogma. *Nat Rev Neurosci. 1*, 67-73.

[17] Kaplan MS. (2001) Environment complexity stimulates visual cortex neurogenesis: death of a dogma and a research career. *Trends Neurosci. 24*, 617-20.

[18] Taupin P, Gage FH. (2002) Adult neurogenesis and neural stem cells of the central nervous system in mammals. *J Neurosci Res. 69*, 745-9.

[19] Miller MW, Nowakowski RS. (1988) Use of bromodeoxyuridine-immunohistochemistry to examine the proliferation, migration and time of origin of cells in the central nervous system. *Brain Res. 457*, 44-52.

[20] Taupin P. (2007) BrdU Immunohistochemistry for Studying Adult Neurogenesis: paradigms, pitfalls, limitations, and validation. *Brain Research Reviews. 53*, 198-214.

[21] Taupin P. (2007) Protocols for Studying Adult Neurogenesis: Insights and Recent Developments. *Regenerative Medicine. 2*, 51-62.

[22] Luskin MB. (1993) Restricted proliferation and migration of postnatally generated neurons derived from the forebrain subventricular zone. *Neuron. 11*, 173-89.

[23] Corotto FS, Henegar JA, Maruniak JA. (1993) Neurogenesis persists in the subependymal layer of the adult mouse brain. *Neurosci Lett. 149*, 111-4.

[24] Lois C, Alvarez-Buylla A. (1994) Long-distance neuronal migration in the adult mammalian brain. *Science. 264*, 1145-8.

[25] Carlen M, Cassidy RM, Brismar H, Smith GA, Enquist LW, Frisen J. (2002) Functional integration of adult-born neurons. *Curr Biol. 12*, 606-8.

[26] Kornack DR, Rakic P. (2001) The generation, migration, and differentiation of olfactory neurons in the adult primate brain. *Proc Natl Acad Sci U S A. 98*, 4752-7.

[27] Pencea V, Bingaman KD, Freedman LJ, Luskin MB. (2001) Neurogenesis in the subventricular zone and rostral migratory stream of the neonatal and adult primate forebrain. *Exp Neurol. 172*, 1-16.

[28] Bedard A, Parent A. (2004) Evidence of newly generated neurons in the human olfactory bulb. Brain Res Dev. *Brain Res. 151*, 159-68.

[29] Curtis MA, Kam M, Nannmark U, Anderson MF, Axell MZ, Wikkelso C, Holtas S, van Roon-Mom WM, Bjork-Eriksson T, Nordborg C, Frisen J, Dragunow M, Faull RL, Eriksson PS. (2007) Human neuroblasts migrate to the olfactory bulb via a lateral ventricular extension. *Science. 315*, 1243-9.

[30] Lois C, Garcia-Verdugo LM, Alvarez-Buylla A. (1996) Chain migration of neuronal precursors. *Science. 271*, 978-81.

[31] Doetsch F, Alvarez-Buylla A. (1996) Network of tangential pathways for neuronal migration in adult mammalian brain. *Proc Natl Acad Sci U S A. 93*, 14895-900.

[32] Sanai N, Tramontin AD, Quinones-Hinojosa A, Barbaro NM, Gupta N, Kunwar S, Lawton MT, McDermott MW, Parsa AT, Garcia-Verdugo JM, Berger MS, Alvarez-Buylla A. (2004) Unique astrocyte ribbon in adult human brain contains neural stem cells but lacks chain migration. *Nature. 427*, 740-4.

[33] Cameron HA, Woolley CS, McEwen BS, Gould E. (1993) Differentiation of newly born neurons and glia in the dentate gyrus of the adult rat. *Neurosci. 56*, 337-44.

[34] Stanfield BB, Trice JE. (1988) Evidence that granule cells generated in the dentate gyrus of adult rats extend axonal projections. *Exp Brain Res. 72*, 399-406.

[35] Markakis EA, Gage FH. (1999) Adult-generated neurons in the dentate gyrus send axonal projections to field CA3 and are surrounded by synaptic vesicles. *J Comp Neurol. 406*, 449-60.

[36] Van Praag H, Schinder AF, Christie BR, Toni N, Palmer TD, Gage FH. (2002) Functional neurogenesis in the adult hippocampus. *Nature. 415*, 1030-4.

[37] Gould E, Reeves AJ, Fallah M, Tanapat P, Gross CG, Fuchs E. (1999) Hippocampal neurogenesis in adult Old World primates. *Proc Natl Acad Sci U S A. 96*, 5263-7.

[38] Kornack DR, Rakic P. (1999) Continuation of neurogenesis in the hippocampus of the adult macaque monkey. *Proc Natl Acad Sci U S A. 96*, 5768-73.

[39] Eriksson PS, Perfilieva E, Bjork-Eriksson T, Alborn AM, Nordborg C, Peterson DA, Gage FH. (1998) Neurogenesis in the adult human hippocampus. *Nat Med. 4*, 1313-7.

[40] Hastings NB, Gould E. (1999) Rapid extension of axons into the CA3 region by adult-generated granule cells. J Comp Neurol. 413, 146-54. Erratum in: (1999) *J Comp Neurol. 415*, 144.

[41] Morshead CM, van der Kooy D. (1992) Postmitotic death is the fate of constitutively proliferating cells in the subependymal layer of the adult mouse brain. *J Neurosci. 12*, 249-56.

[42] Cameron HA, McKay RD. (2001) Adult neurogenesis produces a large pool of new granule cells in the dentate gyrus. *J Comp Neurol. 435*, 406-17.

[43] Kempermann G, Kuhn HG, Gage FH. (1997) More hippocampal neurons in adult mice living in an enriched environment. *Nature. 386*, 493-5.

[44] Rakic P. (1998) Young neurons for old brains? *Nat Neurosci. 1*, 645-7.

[45] Kornack DR, Rakic P. (2001) Cell proliferation without neurogenesis in adult primate neocortex. *Science. 294*, 2127-30.

[46] Rietze R, Poulin P, Weiss S. (2000) Mitotically active cells that generate neurons and astrocytes are present in multiple regions of the adult mouse hippocampus. *J Comp Neurol. 424*, 397-408.

[47] Gould E, Vail N, Wagers M, Gross CG. (2001) Adult-generated hippocampal and neocortical neurons in macaques have a transient existence. *Proc Natl Acad Sci U S A. 98*, 10910-7.

[48] Gould E, Reeves AJ, Graziano MS, Gross CG. (1999) Neurogenesis in the neocortex of adult primates. *Science. 286*, 548-52.

[49] Bedard A, Cossette M, Levesque M, Parent A. (2002) Proliferating cells can differentiate into neurons in the striatum of normal adult monkey. *Neurosci Lett. 328*, 213-6.

[50] Bernier PJ, Bedard A, Vinet J, Levesque M, Parent A. (2002) Newly generated neurons in the amygdala and adjoining cortex of adult primates. *Proc Natl Acad Sci U S A. 99*, 11464-9.

[51] Zhao M, Momma S, Delfani K, Carlen M, Cassidy RM, Johansson CB, Brismar H, Shupliakov O, Frisen J, Janson AM. (2003) Evidence for neurogenesis in the adult mammalian substantia nigra. *Proc Natl Acad Sci U S A. 100*, 7925-30.

[52] Lie DC, Dziewczapolski G, Willhoite AR, Kaspar BK, Shults CW, Gage FH. (2002) The adult substantia nigra contains progenitor cells with neurogenic potential. *J Neurosci. 22*, 6639-49.

[53] Koketsu D, Mikami A, Miyamoto Y, Hisatsune T. (2003) Nonrenewal of neurons in the cerebral neocortex of adult macaque monkeys. *J Neurosci. 23*, 937-42.

[54] Frielingsdorf H, Schwarz K, Brundin P, Mohapel P. (2004) No evidence for new dopaminergic neurons in the adult mammalian substantia nigra. *Proc Natl Acad Sci U S A. 101*, 10177-82.

[55] Doetsch F, Caille I, Lim DA, Garcia-Verdugo JM, Alvarez-Buylla A. (1999) Subventricular zone astrocytes are neural stem cells in the adult mammalian brain. *Cell. 97*, 703-16.

[56] Seri B, Garcia-Verdugo JM, McEwen BS, Alvarez-Buylla A. (2001) Astrocytes give rise to new neurons in the adult mammalian hippocampus. *J Neurosci. 21*, 7153-60.

[57] Filippov V, Kronenberg G, Pivneva T, Reuter K, Steiner B, Wang LP, Yamaguchi M, Kettenmann H, Kempermann G. (2003) Subpopulation of nestin-expressing progenitor cells in the adult murine hippocampus shows electrophysiological and morphological characteristics of astrocytes. *Mol Cell Neurosci. 23*, 373-82.

[58] Garcia-Verdugo JM, Doetsch F, Wichterle H, Lim DA, Alvarez-Buylla A. (1998) Architecture and cell types of the adult subventricular zone: in search of the stem cells. *J Neurobiol. 36*, 234-48.

[59] Morshead CM, Reynolds BA, Craig CG, McBurney MW, Staines WA, Morassutti D, Weiss S, van der Kooy D. (1994) Neural stem cells in the adult mammalian forebrain: a relatively quiescent subpopulation of subependymal cells. *Neuron. 13*, 1071-82.

[60] Doetsch F, Garcia-Verdugo JM, Alvarez-Buylla A. (1999) Regeneration of a germinal layer in the adult mammalian brain. *Proc Natl Acad Sci U S A. 96*, 11619-24.

[61] Seri B, Garcia-Verdugo JM, Collado-Morente L, McEwen BS, Alvarez-Buylla A. (2004) Cell types, lineage, and architecture of the germinal zone in the adult dentate gyrus. *J Comp Neurol. 478*, 359-78. Erratum in: (2004) J Comp Neurol. 480, 427.

[62] Debus E, Weber K, Osborn M. (1983) Monoclonal antibodies specific for glial fibrillary acidic (GFA) protein and for each of the neurofilament triplet polypeptides. *Differentiation. 25*, 193-203.

[63] Lendahl U, Zimmerman LB, McKay RD. (1990) CNS stem cells express a new class of intermediate filament protein. *Cell. 60*, 585-95.

[64] Dahlstrand J, Lardelli M, Lendahl U. (1995) Nestin mRNA expression correlates with the central nervous system progenitor cell state in many, but not all, regions of developing central nervous system. *Brain Res. Dev Brain Res. 84*, 109-29.

[65] Johansson CB, Momma S, Clarke DL, Risling M, Lendahl U, Frisen J. (1999) Identification of a neural stem cell in the adult mammalian central nervous system. *Cell. 96*, 25-34.

[66] Chiasson BJ, Tropepe V, Morshead CM, van der Kooy D. (1999) Adult mammalian forebrain ependymal and subependymal cells demonstrate proliferative potential, but only subependymal cells have neural stem cell characteristics. *J Neurosci. 19*, 4462-71.

[67] Laywell ED, Rakic P, Kukekov VG, Holland EC, Steindler DA. (2000) Identification of a multipotent astrocytic stem cell in the immature and adult mouse brain. *Proc Natl Acad Sci U S A. 97*, 13883-8.

[68] Morshead CM, Garcia AD, Sofroniew MV, van Der Kooy D. (2003) The ablation of glial fibrillary acidic protein-positive cells from the adult central nervous system results in the loss of forebrain neural stem cells but not retinal stem cells. *Eur J Neurosci. 18*, 76-84.

[69] Imura T, Kornblum HI, Sofroniew MV. (2003) The predominant neural stem cell isolated from postnatal and adult forebrain but not early embryonic forebrain expresses GFAP. *J Neurosci. 23*, 2824-32.

[70] Garcia AD, Doan NB, Imura T, Bush TG, Sofroniew MV. (2004) GFAP-expressing progenitors are the principal source of constitutive neurogenesis in adult mouse forebrain. *Nat Neurosci. 7*, 1233-41.

[71] Ribak CE, Seress L. (1983) Five types of basket cell in the hippocampal dentate gyrus: a combined Golgi and electron microscopic study. *J Neurocytol. 12*, 577-97.

[72] Seress L, Ribak CE. (1983) GABAergic cells in the dentate gyrus appear to be local circuit and projection neurons. *Exp Brain Res. 50*, 173-82.

[73] Pinaud R, Velho TA, Jeong JK, Tremere LA, Leao RM, von Gersdorff H, Mello CV. (2004) GABAergic neurons participate in the brain's response to birdsong auditory stimulation. *Eur J Neurosci. 20*, 1318-30.

[74] Davies P, Anderton B, Kirsch J, Konnerth A, Nitsch R, Sheetz M. (1998) First one in, last one out: the role of gabaergic transmission in generation and degeneration. *Prog Neurobiol. 55*, 651-8.

[75] Ben-Ari Y. (2002) Excitatory actions of gaba during development: the nature of the nurture. *Nat Rev Neurosci. 3*, 728-39.

[76] Ben-Ari Y, Tseeb V, Raggozzino D, Khazipov R, Gaiarsa JL. (1994) Gamma-Aminobutyric acid (GABA): a fast excitatory transmitter which may regulate the development of hippocampal neurones in early postnatal life. *Prog Brain Res. 102*, 261-73.

[77] Gaiarsa JL, McLean H, Congar P, Leinekugel X, Khazipov R, Tseeb V, Ben-Ari Y. (1995) Postnatal maturation of gamma-aminobutyric acidA and B-mediated inhibition in the CA3 hippocampal region of the rat. *J Neurobiol. 26*, 339-49.

[78] Lipton SA, Kater SB. (1989) Neurotransmitter regulation of neuronal outgrowth, plasticity and survival. *Trends Neurosci. 12*, 265-70.

[79] Katz LC, Shatz CJ. (1996) Synaptic activity and the construction of cortical circuits, *Science. 274*, 1133-8.

[80] Ben-Ari Y, Khazipov R, Leinekugel X, Caillard O, Gaiarsa JL. (1997) GABAA, NMDA and AMPA receptors: a developmentally regulated 'menage a trois'. *Trends Neurosci. 20*, 523-9.

[81] Owens DF, Kriegstein AR. (2002) Is there more to GABA than synaptic inhibition? *Nat Rev Neurosci. 3*, 715-27.

[82] LoTurco JJ, Owens DF, Heath MJ, Davis MB, Kriegstein AR. (1995) GABA and glutamate depolarize cortical progenitor cells and inhibit DNA synthesis. *Neuron. 15*, 1287-98.

[83] Wang LP, Kempermann G, Kettenmann H. (2005) A subpopulation of precursor cells in the mouse dentate gyrus receives synaptic GABAergic input. *Mol Cell Neurosci. 29*, 181-9.

[84] Tozuka Y, Fukuda S, Namba T, Seki T, Hisatsune T. (2005) GABAergic excitation promotes neuronal differentiation in adult hippocampal progenitor cells. *Neuron. 47*, 803-15.

[85] Wang DD, Krueger DD, Bordey A. (2003) GABA depolarizes neuronal progenitors of the postnatal subventricular zone via GABAA receptor activation. *J Physiol. 550*, 785-800.

[86] Schwab MH, Bartholomae A, Heimrich B, Feldmeyer D, Druffel-Augustin S, Goebbels S, Naya FJ, Zhao S, Frotscher M, Tsai MJ, Nave KA. (2000) Neuronal basic helix-loop-helix proteins (NEX and BETA2/Neuro D) regulate terminal granule cell differentiation in the hippocampus. J Neurosci. 20, 3714-24. Erratum in: (2000) *J Neurosci. 20*, 8227.

[87] Deisseroth K, Singla S, Toda H, Monje M, Palmer TD, Malenka RC. (2004) Excitation-neurogenesis coupling in adult neural stem/progenitor cells. *Neuron. 42*, 535-52.

[88] Ge S, Goh EL, Sailor KA, Kitabatake Y, Ming GL, Song H. (2005) GABA regulates synaptic integration of newly generated neurons in the adult brain. *Nature. 439*, 589-93.

[89] Liu X, Wang Q, Haydar TF, Bordey A. (2005) Nonsynaptic GABA signaling in postnatal subventricular zone controls proliferation of GFAP-expressing progenitors. *Nat Neurosci. 8*, 1179-87.

[90] Bolteus AJ, Bordey A. (2004) GABA release and uptake regulate neuronal precursor migration in the postnatal subventricular zone. *J Neurosci.* 24, 7623-31.

[91] Esposito MS, Piatti VC, Laplagne DA, Morgenstern NA, Ferrari CC, Pitossi FJ, Schinder AF. (2005) Neuronal differentiation in the adult hippocampus recapitulates embryonic development. *J Neurosci. 25*, 10074-86.

[92] Reynolds BA, Weiss S. (1992) Generation of neurons and astrocytes from isolated cells of the adult mammalian central nervous system. *Science. 255*, 1707-10.

[93] Gage FH, Coates PW, Palmer TD, Kuhn HG, Fisher LJ, Suhonen JO, Peterson DA, Suhr ST, Ray J. (1995) Survival and differentiation of adult neuronal progenitor cells transplanted to the adult brain. *Proc Natl Acad Sci U S A. 92*, 11879-83.

[94] Gritti A, Parati EA, Cova L, Frolichsthal P, Galli R, Wanke E, Faravelli L, Morassutti DJ, Roisen F, Nickel DD, Vescovi AL. (1996) Multipotential stem cells from the adult mouse brain proliferate and self-renew in response to basic fibroblast growth factor. *J Neurosci. 16*, 1091-100.

[95] Palmer TD, Takahashi J, Gage FH. (1997) The adult rat hippocampus contains primordial neural stem cells. *Mol Cell Neurosci. 8*, 389-404.

[96] Roy NS, Wang S, Jiang L, Kang J, Benraiss A, Harrison-Restelli C, Fraser RA, Couldwell WT, Kawaguchi A, Okano H, Nedergaard M, Goldman SA. (2000) In vitro

neurogenesis by progenitor cells isolated from the adult human hippocampus. *Nat Med. 6*, 271-7.

[97] Palmer TD, Schwartz PH, Taupin P, Kaspar B, Stein SA, Gage FH. (2001) Cell culture. Progenitor cells from human brain after death. *Nature. 411*, 42-3.

[98] Shihabuddin LS, Horner PJ, Ray J, Gage FH. (2000) Adult spinal cord stem cells generate neurons after transplantation in the adult dentate gyrus. *J Neurosci. 20*, 8727-35.

[99] Seaberg RM, van der Kooy D. (2002) Adult rodent neurogenic regions: the ventricular subependyma contains neural stem cells, but the dentate gyrus contains restricted progenitors. *J Neurosci. 22*, 1784-93.

[100] Bull ND, Bartlett PF. (2005) The adult mouse hippocampal progenitor is neurogenic but not a stem cell. *J Neurosci. 25*, 10815-21.

[101] Yaworsky PJ, Kappen C. (1999) Heterogeneity of neural progenitor cells revealed by enhancers in the nestin gene. *Dev Biol. 205*, 309-21.

[102] Chin VI, Taupin P, Sanga S, Scheel J, Gage FH, Bhatia SN. (2004) Microfabricated platform for studying stem cell fates. *Biotechnol Bioeng. 88*, 399-415.

[103] Taupin, P. (2005) Adult neurogenesis in the mammalian central nervous system: functionality and potential clinical interest. *Med Sci Monit. 11*, RA247-52.

[104] Kuhn HG, Dickinson-Anson H, Gage FH. (1996) Neurogenesis in the dentate gyrus of the adult rat: age-related decrease of neuronal progenitor proliferation. *J Neurosci. 16*, 2027-33.

[105] Gould E, Tanapat P, McEwen BS, Flugge G, Fuchs E. (1998) Proliferation of granule cell precursors in the dentate gyrus of adult monkeys is diminished by stress. *Proc Natl Acad Sci U S A. 95*, 3168-71.

[106] Gould E, Beylin A, Tanapat P, Reeves A, Shors TJ. (1999) Learning enhances adult neurogenesis in the hippocampal formation. *Nat Neurosci. 2*, 260-5.

[107] van Praag H, Kempermann G, Gage FH. (1999) Running increases cell proliferation and neurogenesis in the adult mouse dentate gyrus. *Nat Neurosci. 2*, 266-70.

[108] Parent JM, Yu TW, Leibowitz RT, Geschwind DH, Sloviter RS, Lowenstein DH. (1997) Dentate granule cell neurogenesis is increased by seizures and contributes to aberrant network reorganization in the adult rat hippocampus. *J Neurosci. 17*, 3727-38.

[109] Liu J, Solway K, Messing RO, Sharp FR. (1998) Increased neurogenesis in the dentate gyrus after transient global ischemia in gerbils. *J Neurosci. 18*, 7768-78.

[110] Dash PK, Mach SA, Moore AN. (2001) Enhanced neurogenesis in the rodent hippocampus following traumatic brain injury. *J Neurosci Res. 63*, 313-9.

[111] Curtis MA, Penney EB, Pearson AG, van Roon-Mom WM, Butterworth NJ, Dragunow M, Connor B, Faull RL. (2003) Increased cell proliferation and neurogenesis in the adult human Huntington's disease brain. *Proc Natl Acad Sci U S A. 100*, 9023-7.

[112] Jin K, Peel AL, Mao XO, Xie L, Cottrell BA, Henshall DC, Greenberg DA. (2004) Increased hippocampal neurogenesis in Alzheimer's disease. *Proc Natl Acad Sci U S A. 101*, 343-7.

[113] Shors TJ, Miesegaes G, Beylin A, Zhao M, Rydel T, Gould E. (2001) Neurogenesis in the adult is involved in the formation of trace memories. *Nature. 410*, 372-6. Erratum in: (2001) *Nature. 414*, 938.

[114] Santarelli L, Saxe M, Gross C, Surget A, Battaglia F, Dulawa S, Weisstaub N, Lee J, Duman R, Arancio O, Belzung C, Hen R. (2003) Requirement of hippocampal neurogenesis for the behavioral effects of antidepressants. *Science. 301*, 805-9.

[115] Snyder JS, Hong NS, McDonald RJ, Wojtowicz JM. (2005) A role for adult neurogenesis in spatial long-term memory. *Neurosci. 130*, 843-52.

[116] Rhodes JS, van Praag H, Jeffrey S, Girard I, Mitchell GS, Garland T. Jr, Gage FH. (2003) Exercise increases hippocampal neurogenesis to high levels but does not improve spatial learning in mice bred for increased voluntary wheel running. *Behav Neurosci. 117*, 1006-16. Erratum in: (2003) Behav Neurosci. 118, 305.

[117] Leuner B, Mendolia-Loffredo S, Kozorovitskiy Y, Samburg D, Gould E, Shors TJ. (2004) Learning enhances the survival of new neurons beyond the time when the hippocampus is required for memory. *J Neurosci. 24*, 7477-81.

[118] Dupret D, Montaron MF, Drapeau E, Aurousseau C, Le Moal M, Piazza PV, Abrous DN. (2005) Methylazoxymethanol acetate does not fully block cell genesis in the young and aged dentate gyrus. *Eur J Neurosci. 22*, 778-83.

[119] Nestler EJ, Barrot M, DiLeone RJ, Eisch AJ, Gold SJ, Monteggia LM. (2002) Neurobiology of depression. *Neuron. 34*, 13-25.

[120] Ebmeier KP, Donaghey C, Steele JD. (2006) Recent developments and current controversies in depression. *Lancet. 367*, 153-67.

[121] Taupin P. (2006) Neurogenesis and the Effects of Antidepressants. *Drug Target Insights. 1*, 13-7.

[122] Arvidsson A, Collin T, Kirik D, Kokaia Z, Lindvall O. (2002) Neuronal replacement from endogenous precursors in the adult brain after stroke. *Nat Med. 8*, 963-70.

[123] Jin K, Sun Y, Xie L, Peel A, Mao XO, Batteur S, Greenberg DA. (2003) Directed migration of neuronal precursors into the ischemic cerebral cortex and striatum. *Mol Cell Neurosci. 24*, 171-89.

[124] Carpentier P, Delamanche IS, Le Bert M, Blanchet G, Bouchaud C. (1990) Seizure-related opening of the blood-brain barrier induced by soman: possible correlation with the acute neuropathology observed in poisoned rats. *Neurotoxicology*. 11, 493-508.

[125] Sharma HS, Cervos-Navarro J, Dey PK. (1991) Increased blood-brain barrier permeability following acute short-term swimming exercise in conscious normotensive young rats. *Neurosci Res. 10*, 211-21.

[126] Herrup K, Arendt T. (2002) Re-expression of cell cycle proteins induces neuronal cell death during Alzheimer's disease. *J Alzheimers Dis. 4*, 243-7.

[127] Herrup K, Neve R, Ackerman SL, Copani A. (2004) Divide and die: cell cycle events as triggers of nerve cell death. *J Neurosci. 24*, 9232-9.

[128] Kuan CY, Schloemer AJ, Lu A, Burns KA, Weng WL, Williams MT, Strauss KI, Vorhees CV, Flavell RA, Davis RJ, Sharp FR, Rakic P. (2004) Hypoxia-ischemia induces DNA synthesis without cell proliferation in dying neurons in adult rodent brain. *J Neurosci. 24*, 10763-72.

[129] Yang Y, Geldmacher DS, Herrup K. (2001) DNA replication precedes neuronal cell death in Alzheimer's disease. *J Neurosci. 21*, 2661-8.

[130] Yang Y, Mufson EJ, Herrup K. (2003) Neuronal cell death is preceded by cell cycle events at all stages of Alzheimer's disease. *J Neurosci. 23*, 2557-63.

[131] Morris SM. (1991) The genetic toxicology of 5-bromodeoxyuridine in mammalian cells. *Mutat Res. 258*, 161-88.

[132] Sekerkova G, Ilijic E, Mugnaini E. (2004) Bromodeoxyuridine administered during neurogenesis of the projection neurons causes cerebellar defects in rat. *J Comp Neurol. 470*, 221-39.

[133] Caldwell MA, He X, Svendsen CN. (2005) 5-Bromo-2'-deoxyuridine is selectively toxic to neuronal precursors in vitro. *Eur J Neurosci. 22*, 2965-70.

[134] Kaplan MS. (1988) Plasticity after brain lesions: contemporary concepts. *Arch Phys Med Rehabil. 69*, 984-91.

[135] Taupin P. (2006) Adult neurogenesis and neuroplasticity. *Restor Neurol Neurosci. 24*, 9-15.

[136] Ourednik J, Ourednik V, Lynch WP, Schachner M, Snyder EY. (2002) Neural stem cells display an inherent mechanism for rescuing dysfunctional neurons. *Nat Biotechnol. 20*, 1103-10.

[137] Bjugstad KB, Redmond DE Jr, Teng YD, Elsworth JD, Roth RH, Blanchard BC, Snyder EY, Sladek JR Jr. (2005) Neural stem cells implanted into MPTP-treated monkeys increase the size of endogenous tyrosine hydroxylase-positive cells found in the striatum: a return to control measures. *Cell Transplant. 14*, 183-92.

[138] Pfeifer K, Vroemen M, Blesch A, Weidner N. (2004) Adult neural progenitor cells provide a permissive guiding substrate for corticospinal axon growth following spinal cord injury. *Eur J Neurosci. 20*, 1695-704.

[139] Park KI, Teng YD, Snyder EY. (2002) The injured brain interacts reciprocally with neural stem cells supported by scaffolds to reconstitute lost tissue. *Nat Biotechnol. 20*, 1111-7.

[140] Pluchino S, Zanotti L, Rossi B, Brambilla E, Ottoboni L, Salani G, Martinello M, Cattalini A, Bergami A, Furlan R, Comi G, Constantin G, Martino G. (2005) Neurosphere-derived multipotent precursors promote neuroprotection by an immunomodulatory mechanism. *Nature. 436*, 266-71.

[141] Cummings BJ, Uchida N, Tamaki SJ, Salazar DL, Hooshmand M, Summer R, Gage FH, Anderson AJ. (2005) Human neural stem cells differentiate and promote locomotor recovery in spinal cord-injured mice. *Proc Natl Acad Sci U S A. 102*, 14069-74.

[142] Taupin P. (2006) Autologous transplantation in the central nervous system. *Indian Journal of Medical Research. 124*, 613-8.

[143] Taupin P. (2006) Neural Progenitor and Stem Cells in the Adult Central Nervous System. *Annals, Academy of Medicine, Singapore. 35*, 814-7.

[144] Brown J, Cooper-Kuhn CM, Kempermann G, Van Praag H, Winkler J, Gage FH, Kuhn HG. (2003) Enriched environment and physical activity stimulate hippocampal but not olfactory bulb neurogenesis. *Eur J Neurosci. 17*, 2042-6.

[145] Ra SM, Kim H, Jang MH, Shin MC, Lee TH, Lim BV, Kim CJ, Kim EH, Kim KM, Kim SS. (2002) Treadmill running and swimming increase cell proliferation in the hippocampal dentate gyrus of rats. *Neurosci Lett. 333*, 123-6.

[146] Nixon K, Crews FT. (2002) Binge ethanol exposure decreases neurogenesis in adult rat hippocampus. *J Neurochem. 83*, 1087-93.

[147] Herrera DG, Yague AG, Johnsen-Soriano S, Bosch-Morell F, Collado-Morente L, Muriach M, Romero FJ, Garcia-Verdugo JM. (2003) Selective impairment of hippocampal neurogenesis by chronic alcoholism, protective effects of an antioxidant. *Proc Natl Acad Sci U S A. 100*, 7919-24.

[148] Rice AC, Bullock MR, Shelton KL. (2004) Chronic ethanol consumption transiently reduces adult neural progenitor cell proliferation. *Brain Res. 1011*, 94-8.

[149] Lee J, Duan W, Long JM, Ingram DK, Mattson MP. (2000) Dietary restriction increases the number of newly generated neural cells, and induces BDNF expression, in the dentate gyrus of rats. *J Mol Neurosci.15*, 99-108.

[150] Lee J, Seroogy KB, Mattson MP. (2002) Dietary restriction enhances neurotrophin expression and neurogenesis in the hippocampus of adult mice. J Neurochem. 80, 539-47.

[151] Mirescu C, Peters JD, Gould E. (2004) Early life experience alters response of adult neurogenesis to stress. *Nat Neurosci. 7*, 841-6.

[152] Lu L, Bao G, Chen H, Xia P, Fan X, Zhang J, Pei G, Ma L. (2003) Modification of hippocampal neurogenesis and neuroplasticity by social environments. *Exp Neurol. 183*, 600-9.

[153] Malberg JE, Duman RS. (2003) Cell proliferation in adult hippocampus is decreased by inescapable stress, reversal by fluoxetine treatment. *Neuropsychopharmacology. 28*, 1562-71.

[154] Kuhn HG, Dickinson-Anson H, Gage FH. (1996) Neurogenesis in the dentate gyrus of the adult rat, age-related decrease of neuronal progenitor proliferation. *J Neurosci. 16*, 2027-33.

[155] Tropepe V, Craig CG, Morshead CM, van der Kooy D. (1997) Transforming growth factor-alpha null and senescent mice show decreased neural progenitor cell proliferation in the forebrain subependyma. *J Neurosci. 17*, 7850-9.

[156] Enwere E, Shingo T, Gregg C, Fujikawa H, Ohta S, Weiss S. (2004) Aging results in reduced epidermal growth factor receptor signaling, diminished olfactory neurogenesis, and deficits in fine olfactory discrimination. *J Neurosci. 24*, 8354-65.

[157] Tanapat P, Hastings NB, Reeves AJ, Gould E. (1999) Estrogen stimulates a transient increase in the number of new neurons in the dentate gyrus of the adult female rat. *J Neurosci. 19*, 5792-801.

[158] Smith MT, Pencea V, Wang Z, Luskin MB, Insel TR. (2001) Increased number of BrdU-labeled neurons in the rostral migratory stream of the estrous prairie vole. *Horm Behav. 39*, 11-21.

[159] Feng R, Rampon C, Tang YP, Shrom D, Jin J, Kyin M, Sopher B, Miller MW, Ware CB, Martin GM, Kim SH, Langdon RB, Sisodia SS, Tsien JZ. (2001) Deficient neurogenesis in forebrain-specific presenilin-1 knockout mice is associated with reduced clearance of hippocampal memory traces. *Neuron. 32*, 911-26. Erratum in: (2002) *Neuron. 33*, 313.

[160] Jin K, Galvan V, Xie L, Mao XO, Gorostiza OF, Bredesen DE, Greenberg DA. (2004) Enhanced neurogenesis in Alzheimer's disease transgenic (PDGF-APPSw,Ind) mice. *Proc Natl Acad Sci U S A. 101*, 13363-7.

[161] Covolan L, Ribeiro LT, Longo BM, Mello LE. (2000) Cell damage and neurogenesis in the dentate granule cell layer of adult rats after pilocarpine- or kainate-induced status epilepticus. *Hippocampus. 10*, 69-80.

[162] Gray WP, Sundstrom LE. (1998) Kainic acid increases the proliferation of granule cell progenitors in the dentate gyrus of the adult rat. *Brain Res. 790*, 52-9.

[163] Bengzon J, Kokaia Z, Elmer E, Nanobashvili A, Kokaia M, Lindvall O. (1997) Apoptosis and proliferation of dentate gyrus neurons after single and intermittent limbic seizures. *Proc Natl Acad Sci U S A. 94*, 10432-7.

Chapter X

PHYSIO- AND PATHOLOGY

ABSTRACT

The hippocampus is involved in physio- and pathological processes, like learning and memory, Alzheimer's disease (AD) and epilepsy. The mechanisms underlying these processes remain mostly unknown. With the recent confirmation that neurogenesis occurs in the adult brain, and particularly in the hippocampus, researchers are aiming to understand the involvement and contribution of newly generated neuronal cells in the adult brain to the physio- and pathology of the central nervous system (CNS), and particularly the hippocampus.

INTRODUCTION

The hippocampus lies beneath the neocortex, on the basal medial surface of the temporal lobe [1]. It is a key region of the cerebral cortex involved in learning and memory [2,3]. Though the precise role of the hippocampus in learning and memory is yet to be fully determined, it is widely accepted that the hippocampus plays an essential role in the formation of new memories and spatial information processing [4,5]. In 1966, Terge Lomo discovered long-term potentiation (LTP), a lasting increase in synaptic strength and transmission [6]. This form of synaptic plasticity, specific to the hippocampus, is believed to be a mechanism through which memories are formed [7]. The hippocampus is one of the first regions of the brain to be affected in Alzheimer's disease, a neurodegenerative disease. This underlies the early memory impairments associated with the disease [8,9]. The hippocampus is also one of the regions critical in the pathology of epilepsy [10]. Despite significant progresses made in the understanding of these physio- and pathological processes, their molecular and cellular mechanisms remain mostly unknown [11].

Over the past decade, the confirmation that the hippocampus along with the subventricular zone (SVZ) are the two main regions of the adult brain where neurogenesis occurs in mammals, including in humans, raises the question of the involvement of newly generated neuronal cells in the physio- and pathology of the CNS, and particularly the hippocampus [12-16].

Learning and Memory

The first reports that neurogenesis in the adult hippocampus may be involved in learning and memory came from studies conducted by Gould et al. (1999) and van Praag et al. (1999). Gould et al. (1999) reported that hippocampal neurogenesis is enhanced in response to training on the Morris water maze task, an associative learning task that requires the hippocampus [17]. Reciprocally, van Praag et al. (1999) reported that increased hippocampal neurogenesis, in mice submitted to environmental enrichment -wheel running-, is correlated with improved performance in the Morris water maze task [18].

Other studies reveal that alteration of hippocampal neurogenesis, using anti-mitotic treatments or brain irradiation, reveals that neurogenesis is involved in the formation of memory dependent of the hippocampus, like the formation of trace memories and short-term memory, but not all forms of hippocampal-dependent memory [19-21]. Low-dose whole-brain X-ray irradiation inhibits adult hippocampal neurogenesis [22]. More recently, a study with Ames dwarf mice shows that these adult mice elicit a higher rate of hippocampal neurogenesis compared to normal mice [23]. Ames dwarf mice are a strain of mice that lives considerably longer than normal mice and maintain physiological functions at youthful levels including cognitive functions. These mice also have a level of insulin growth factor-I (IGF-I) protein that is upregulated in the hippocampus [23]. These results suggest that local/hippocampal IGF-I, known to regulate hippocampal neurogenesis [24-26], may induce an increase in hippocampal neurogenesis. This increase in hippocampal neurogenesis may contribute to the maintenance of youthful levels of cognitive functions during aging, in these long-lived animals.

Altogether, these data provide strong arguments in favor of a role of adult neurogenesis in learning and memory, and IGF-I may be a key factor in learning and memory associated with neurogenesis.

The involvement of adult neurogenesis in learning and memory has been challenged by other studies. On the one hand, increased hippocampal neurogenesis occurs without improvement of learning and memory performances, in the Morris water maze test, in mice selectively bred for high levels of wheel running [27]. The contribution of adult neurogenesis to the formation of trace memory remains for months and beyond the time required for the retention of trace memories [28]. On the other hand, rodents submitted to hippocampus-dependent learning in the Morris water maze, after the maximal period of newborn cell death show a significant decrease in newly generated neuronal cells in the dentate gyrus (DG) [29]. This suggests that learning may reduce hippocampal neurogenesis, and the effect of learning on neurogenesis may depend on the elapsing time between mitosis and learning.

Studies reveal that adult neurogenesis is involved in LTP, a model believed to be a mechanism through which memories are formed [30]. Hippocampal neurogenesis is stimulated following induction of LTP and a low dose of gamma radiation applied to the brain, that reduces neurogenesis, selectively blocks the induction of LTP in hippocampal slices [31,32]. Other studies show that associative LTP can be induced more easily in young neurons than in mature neurons under identical conditions [33]. These results suggest that newborn neuronal cells in the hippocampus may play a significant role in synaptic plasticity and that newly generated neurons express unique mechanisms to facilitate synaptic plasticity, which may be important for the formation of new memories.

Altogether these data show that there is compelling evidences that hippocampal neurogenesis is involved in some forms of learning and memory and synaptic plasticity. However, the extent of the involvement of newly generated neuronal cells, its underlying mechanisms and interaction with other forms of plasticity in the learning and memory remain to be understood [34].

ALZHEIMER'S DISEASE

Alzheimer's disease (AD) is a form of dementia. It is characterized by progressive cognitive and behavioral impairments. The patient loses first his short-term memory. As the disease progresses, the deficits extend to other forms of cognitive deficits and physical impairments. AD is a neurodegenerative disease, associated initially with a loss of nerve cells in areas of the brain that are vital to memory and other mental abilities, like the hippocampus. As the disease expands, other regions of the brain, particularly of the limbic system, are affected [35]. AD can strike younger people, under age 65. The early-onset form of the disease (EOAD) is primarily genetic of origin and inherited. It is a very rare form of the disease, referred as familial form of AD when inherited. The late-onset (LOAD), over age 65, is not inherited and is the most common type of dementia among older people. It is also referred to as sporadic form of AD. About 3 percent of men and women ages 65 to 74 have AD, and nearly half of those age 85 and older may have the disease. On average, AD patients live from 8 to 10 years after they are diagnosed, though the disease can last for as many as 20 years [35].

AD is characterized by amyloid plaque deposits and neurofibrillary tangles [36,37]. Mutations in three genes, presenilin 1 (PSEN 1), PSEN 2 and amyloid precursor protein (APP), have been identified as causes of EOAD, i.e. familial form of AD [35]. The origin of the non-inherited form of the disease remains unknown; risk factors include expression of different forms of the gene apolipoprotein E (ApoE) and reduced expression of neuronal sortilin-related receptor (SORL1) [38-40]. ApoE is a lipid transport protein localized in the senile or amyloid plaques and neurofibrillary tangles that promotes the formation of amyloid [41-44]. SORL1 belongs to a family of proteins termed retromer, involved in intracellular sorting and trafficking [45]. SORL 1 is involved in the trafficking and recycling of APP [40]. There is currently no cure for AD. Actual treatments consist of drug therapy, and physical support and assistance [35].

Studies from autopsies of AD brain patients reveal that expression of markers for immature neuronal cells, like doublecortin and polysialylated nerve cell adhesion molecule, is increased in the subgranular zone (SGZ) and granular layer of the DG, suggesting that neurogenesis is enhanced in the hippocampus of patients suffering of AD [46]. Adult neurogenesis has been characterized in animal models of AD, like gene altered mice, knockout mice or mice expressing mutant forms of PSEN 1 or APP. Neurogenesis is negatively regulated in the DG and SVZ of knock-out mice for PSEN 1 and APP [47,48], and positively regulated in the DG of transgenic mice expressing the Swedish and Indiana APP mutations, a mutant form of human APP [49] (table 1, chapter 9). The DG and SVZ are the two main regions of the brain where neurogenesis occurs in the adult, including in human [12,15,16]. These animal studies were performed using bromodeoxyurine (5-bromo-2'-deoxyuridine, BrdU) labeling.

BrdU is a thymidine analog that incorporates into the DNA of dividing cells during the S-phase of the cell cycle, and is used for birthdating cells and monitoring cell proliferation [50,51]. The discrepancies between the studies could be explained by the limitation of the transgenic animal models as representative of complex diseases and to study adult phenotypes, like adult neurogenesis [52,53]. Particularly, mutant or deficient mice for single genes, like PSEN 1 and APP, may not fully reproduce the features of AD, associated with loss of multiple cell types. Four to 10% of nerve cells in regions in which degeneration occurs in AD, like the hippocampus, are tetraploids [54]. Nerve cells may have entered the cell cycle and undergone DNA replication, and not completed the cell cycle. It is proposed that cell cycle re-entry, as prelude to apoptosis, and DNA duplication without cell division precedes neuronal death in degenerating regions of the CNS [55]. As BrdU incorporates DNA of dividing cells during the S-phase of the cell cycle, BrdU labeling will not allow discriminate cell proliferation versus abortive cell cycle re-entry and DNA duplication without cell division [56-61]. The existence of aneuploid cells may account for some of the newly generated neuronal cells observed, when using BrdU-labeling in experimental models of AD [62].

In all, though reports suggest that neurogenesis is enhanced in AD. This remains to be further confirmed in the light of recent data showing the occurrence of abortive cell cycle re-entry and the existence of tetraploid cells in regions in which degeneration occurs in AD, particularly the hippocampus.

EPILEPSY

Epilepsy is a brain disorder in which populations of nerve cells signal abnormally. In the individual this translates into a variety of seizures, ranging from mild change in behavior to more severe convulsions, muscles spasm and loss of consciousness [63]. Long-term deficits and impairments in learning, memory and behavior have also been reported [64]. Most seizures originate from illness to brain, like abnormal brain development or injuries, and do not cause brain damage.

Epilepsy is one of the most prevalent neurological disorders, afflicting 0.5 to 1.0 % of the world's population. One of the most common forms of epilepsy is the temporal lobe epilepsy (TLE). Temporal lobe epilepsy often has its onset during childhood or is associated with a prolonged seizure episode early in life that is followed, after a variable latent period, by the development of epilepsy. Treatments are available for epileptic patients. Seizures can be controlled in most cases by modern medicine and surgical removal of seizure-producing areas of the brain [65,66]. Deep brain stimulation is currently investigated for the treatment of certain forms of epilepsy [67].

The hippocampal formation is a critical area in the etiology of epilepsy [68]. It is proposed that the DG may function as a gate, controlling the propagation of seizures [69,70]. Granule cells regulate the throughput of epileptiform activity transiting through the hippocampal formation, by virtue of specific feed forward inhibitory pathways [71]. Autopsies from patients suffering from TLE reveal that the hippocampal formation is preserved, with a dispersed granule cell layer [72,73]. Neuronal cell death in the granular and pyramidal cell layers has been reported in patients suffering from TLE, with granule cell loss occurring at a lesser rate than other hippocampal areas [73]. Ectopic granule-like cells, as defined by the expression of calcium-binding protein or calbindin D28K, are found in the *hilus* and inner molecular layer [72]. The dentate granule cells give rise to abnormal axonal projections to the supragranular inner molecular layer of the DG and the basal dendrites of CA3 pyramidal cells in *stratum oriens*, a process referred as mossy fiber (MF) sprouting [74-76].

It is hypothesized that a reduction in inhibition by loss of interneurons [77] and/or the development of recurrent excitatory circuitry by the sprouting of MFs into ectopic positions, and subsequent hippocampal hyper excitability, are determining events in the pathogenesis of limbic epilepsies [76,78,79]. Alternatively, it has been proposed that aberrant granule cell axonal projections stabilize the network by preferentially innervating inhibitory interneurons, and thereby restoring recurrent inhibition [80]. The implication of MF sprouting in seizures has been challenge by recent data showing that spontaneous recurrent seizures are still observed when MF sprouting is prevented, after pretreatment with the protein synthesis inhibitor cycloheximide, in experimental animal models, like pilocarpine- or kainate-treated animals [81,82]. This shows that the etiology of epilepsy, and particularly the implication of MF sprouting in the pathogenesis of epilepsy, remains to be fully understood.

With the advent in adult neurogenesis and neural stem cells research, investigators have aimed at characterizing the involvement of newborn neuronal cells in the etiology of epilepsy. Using BrdU labeling in adult rodents, research reports show that neurogenesis is enhanced bilaterally in the DG and ectopic granule-like cells BrdU-labeled are detected in the *hilus*, as far as the *Cornu Ammonis* (CA) region CA3, following experimental limbic-induced seizures, like after pilocarpine treatment, perforant path stimulation and kainic acid induced seizures [83-87]. Time course studies reveal that ectopic granule-like cells in the hilus originate from newly generated neuronal cells born in the SGZ. These studies also show that increase of neurogenesis in the DG follows the same time course than MF remodeling, of approximately 1 month [88,89]. This latter observation suggests that MF sprouting may derive from newly born granule-like cells in the DG rather than from preexisting mature dentate granule cells, as previously hypothesized [74-76,90-93].

Low-dose whole-brain X ray-irradiation inhibits adult hippocampal neurogenesis [22]. Low-dose radiation treatment in adult rats, after pilocarpine-induced seizures, does not prevent the induction of seizures and MF sprouting [94,95]. This shows that, although the ectopic granule-like cells are a prominent feature of the response to seizures and originate from newly generated neuronal cells born in the SGZ, newly generated ectopic granule-like are not critical to epileptogenesis. This also shows that MF reorganization arises primarily from mature granule cells and not from newly generated neuronal cells, as previously suggested [83].

Although these data provide a strong argument against a critical role of adult neurogenesis in epileptogenesis, it could be a contributing factor, when present. Altogether these data show that the contribution of adult neurogenesis, ectopic granule-like cells and MF sprouting to epileptogenesis remains to be fully understood.

Conclusion

The hippocampus is a brain region involved in various physio- and pathological processes, like learning and memory, AD and epilepsy. The hippocampus is also a region where neurogenesis occurs throughout adulthood. The mechanisms underlying learning and memory, AD and epilepsy remain mostly unknown, and researchers have aimed to identify the involvement of adult neurogenesis in these processes. Hippocampal neurogenesis is modulated in response to learning and memory tasks involving the hippocampus, in patients with AD and animal models of AD, and epilepsy. This suggests that neurogenesis is involved in these physio- and pathological processes.

Further analysis confirmed this involvement, but the extent and contribution of neurogenesis to these processes remain to be determined. However, limitations of protocols used to study neurogenesis in animal models, like BrdU labeling and transgenic mice, and the difficulty in assessing neurogenesis in human tissue samples, limit not only the investigations, but may lead to false or mis-interpretations of the data observed.

Rigorous investigations complemented with other modes of investigations of adult neurogenesis and newly generated neuronal cells, like the use of retroviruses and the generation of conditional genetically altered mice, will provide invaluable information to study the role of newborn neuronal cells in the physio- pathology of the adult brain, and particularly the hippocampus, in experimental models. In humans, most of these strategies are not applicable, or like BrdU labeling limited to the cases when patients treated with BrdU to trace cancer development, donated tissue samples for research investigations [12,16]. Alternative strategies have recently been used to study neurogenesis in humans, like retrospective birth dating using [14C] [96,97]. This latter strategy may provide an additional means to study the role of neurogenesis in humans.

Addendum

At the time of publication of this manuscript, a report by Reiman et al. (2004) reported the identification of a new gene involved in AD, the gene GAB2. GAB2 normally prevents the formation of Alzheimer's-related neurofibrillary tangles. But certain mutations in GAB2 gene have the opposite effect, making AD more likely [98].

REFERENCES

[1] Squire LR, Stark CE, Clark RE. (2004) The medial temporal lobe. *Annu Rev Neurosci. 27*, 279-306.

[2] Squire LR. (2004) Memory systems of the brain: a brief history and current perspective. *Neurobiol Learn Mem. 82*, 171-7.

[3] Miyashita Y. (2004) Cognitive memory: cellular and network machineries and their top-down control. *Science. 306*, 435-40.

[4] Eichenbaum H. (2004) Hippocampus: cognitive processes and neural representations that underlie declarative memory. *Neuron. 44*, 109-20.

[5] Sweatt JD. (2004) Hippocampal function in cognition. *Psychopharmacology (Berl). 174*, 99-110.

[6] Lomo T. (2003) The discovery of long-term potentiation. *Philos Trans R Soc Lond B Biol Sci. 358*, 617-20.

[7] Malenka RC, Nicoll RA. (1999) Long-term potentiation--a decade of progress? *Science. 285*, 1870-4.

[8] Panegyres PK. (2004) The contribution of the study of neurodegenerative disorders to the understanding of human memory. *QJM. 97*, 555-67.

[9] Lucas JA. (2005) Disorders of memory. *Psychiatr Clin North Am. 28*, 581-97.

[10] Sloviter RS. (2005) The neurobiology of temporal lobe epilepsy: too much information, not enough knowledge. *C R Biol. 328*, 143-53.

[11] Kandel ER. (2001) The molecular biology of memory storage: a dialogue between genes and synapses. *Science. 294*, 1030-8.

[12] Eriksson PS, Perfilieva E, Bjork-Eriksson T, Alborn AM, Nordborg C, Peterson DA, Gage FH. (1998) Neurogenesis in the adult human hippocampus. *Nat Med. 4*, 1313-7.

[13] Gross CG. (2000) Neurogenesis in the adult brain: death of a dogma. *Nat Rev Neurosci. 1*, 67-73.

[14] Kaplan MS. (2001) Environment complexity stimulates visual cortex neurogenesis: death of a dogma and a research career. *Trends Neurosci. 24*, 617-20.

[15] Taupin P, Gage FH. (2002) Adult neurogenesis and neural stem cells of the central nervous system in mammals. *J Neurosci Res. 69*, 745-9.

[16] Curtis MA, Kam M, Nannmark U, Anderson MF, Axell MZ, Wikkelso C, Holtas S, van Roon-Mom WM, Bjork-Eriksson T, Nordborg C, Frisen J, Dragunow M, Faull RL, riksson PS. (2007) Human neuroblasts migrate to the olfactory bulb via a lateral ventricular extension. *Science. 315*, 1243-9.

[17] Gould E, Beylin A, Tanapat P, Reeves A, Shors TJ. (1999) Learning enhances adult neurogenesis in the hippocampal formation. *Nat Neurosci. 2*, 260-5.

[18] van Praag H, Kempermann G, Gage FH. (1999) Running increases cell proliferation and neurogenesis in the adult mouse dentate gyrus. *Nat Neurosci. 2*, 266-70.

[19] Shors TJ, Miesegaes G, Beylin A, Zhao M, Rydel T, Gould E. (2001) Neurogenesis in the adult is involved in the formation of trace memories. *Nature. 410*, 372-6. Erratum in: (2001) *Nature. 414*, 938.

[20] Shors TJ, Townsend DA, Zhao M, Kozorovitskiy Y, Gould E. (2002) Neurogenesis may relate to some but not all types of hippocampal-dependent learning. *Hippocampus. 12*, 578-84.

[21] Madsen TM, Kristjansen PE, Bolwig TG, Wortwein G. (2003) Arrested neuronal proliferation and impaired hippocampal function following fractionated brain irradiation in the adult rat. *Neurosci. 119*, 635-42.

[22] Tada E, Parent JM, Lowenstein DH, Fike JR. (2000) X-irradiation causes a prolonged reduction in cell proliferation in the dentate gyrus of adult rats. *Neurosci. 99*, 33-41.

[23] Sun LY, Evans MS, Hsieh J, Panici J, Bartke A. (2005) Increased neurogenesis in dentate gyrus of long-lived Ames dwarf mice. *Endocrinology. 146*, 1138-44.

[24] Aberg MA, Aberg ND, Hedbacker H, Oscarsson J, Eriksson PS. (2000) Peripheral infusion of IGF-I selectively induces neurogenesis in the adult rat hippocampus. *J Neurosci. 20*, 2896-903.

[25] Arsenijevic Y, Villemure JG, Brunet JF, Bloch JJ, Deglon N, Kostic C, Zurn A, Aebischer P. (2001) Isolation of multipotent neural precursors residing in the cortex of the adult human brain. *Exp Neurol. 170*, 48-62.

[26] Aberg MA, Aberg ND, Palmer TD, Alborn AM, Carlsson-Skwirut C, Bang P, Rosengren LE, Olsson T, Gage FH, Eriksson PS. (2003) IGF-I has a direct proliferative effect in adult hippocampal progenitor cells. *Mol Cell Neurosci. 24*, 23-40.

[27] Rhodes JS, van Praag H, Jeffrey S, Girard I, Mitchell GS, Garland T Jr, Gage FH. (2003) Exercise increases hippocampal neurogenesis to high levels but does not improve spatial learning in mice bred for increased voluntary wheel running. *Behav Neurosci. 117*, 1006-16. Erratum in: (2003) Behav Neurosci. 118, 305.

[28] Leuner B, Mendolia-Loffredo S, Kozorovitskiy Y, Samburg D, Gould E, Shors TJ. (2004) Learning enhances the survival of new neurons beyond the time when the hippocampus is required for memory. *J Neurosci. 24*, 7477-81.

[29] Ambrogini P, Orsini L, Mancini C, Ferri P, Ciaroni S, Cuppini R. (2004) Learning may reduce neurogenesis in adult rat dentate gyrus. *Neurosci Lett. 359*, 13-6.

[30] Bliss TV, Lomo T. (1973) Long-lasting potentiation of synaptic transmission in the dentate area of the anaesthetized rabbit following stimulation of the perforant path. *J Physiol. 232*, 331-56.

[31] van Praag H, Christie BR, Sejnowski TJ, Gage FH. (1999) Running enhances neurogenesis, learning, and long-term potentiation in mice. *Proc Natl Acad Sci U S A. 96*, 13427-31.

[32] Snyder JS, Kee N, Wojtowicz JM. (2001) Effects of adult neurogenesis on synaptic plasticity in the rat dentate gyrus. *J Neurophysiol. 85*, 2423-31.

[33] Schmidt-Hieber C, Jonas P, Bischofberger J. (2004) Enhanced synaptic plasticity in newly generated granule cells of the adult hippocampus. *Nature. 429*, 184-7.

[34] Leuner B, Gould E, Shors TJ. (2006) Is there a link between adult neurogenesis and learning? *Hippocampus. 16*, 216-24.

[35] Caselli RJ, Beach TG, Yaari R, Reiman EM. (2006) Alzheimer's disease a century later. *J Clin Psychiatry. 67*, 1784-800.

[36] Fukutani Y, Kobayashi K, Nakamura I, Watanabe K, Isaki K, Cairns NJ. (1995) Neurons, intracellular and extracellular neurofibrillary tangles in subdivisions of the

hippocampal cortex in normal ageing and Alzheimer's disease. *Neurosci Lett. 200*, 57-60.

[37] Hardy J, Selkoe DJ. (2002) The amyloid hypothesis of Alzheimer's disease: progress and problems on the road to therapeutics. Science. 297, 353-6. Erratum in: (2002) *Science. 297*, 2209.

[38] Corder EH, Saunders AM, Strittmatter WJ, Schmechel DE, Gaskell PC, Small GW, Roses AD, Haines JL, Pericak-Vance MA. (1993) Gene dose of apolipoprotein E type 4 allele and the risk of Alzheimer's disease in late onset families. *Science. 261*, 921-3.

[39] Raber J, Huang Y, Ashford JW. (2004) ApoE genotype accounts for the vast majority of AD risk and AD pathology. *Neurobiol Aging. 25*, 641-50.

[40] Rogaeva E, Meng Y, Lee JH, Gu Y, Kawarai T, Zou F, Katayama T, Baldwin CT, Cheng R, Hasegawa H, Chen F, Shibata N, Lunetta KL, Pardossi-Piquard R, Bohm C, Wakutani Y, Cupples LA, Cuenco KT, Green RC, Pinessi L, Rainero I, Sorbi S, Bruni A, Duara R, Friedland RP, Inzelberg R, Hampe W, Bujo H, Song YQ, Andersen OM, Willnow TE, Graff-Radford N, Petersen RC, Dickson D, Der SD, Fraser PE, Schmitt-Ulms G, Younkin S, Mayeux R, Farrer LA, St George-Hyslop P. (2007) The neuronal sortilin-related receptor SORL1 is genetically associated with Alzheimer disease. *Nat Genet. 39*, 168-77.

[41] Mahley RW. (1988) Apolipoprotein E: cholesterol transport protein with expanding role in cell biology. *Science. 240*, 622-30.

[42] Strittmatter WJ, Saunders AM, Schmechel D, Pericak-Vance M, Enghild J, Salvesen GS, Roses AD. (1993) Apolipoprotein E: high-avidity binding to beta-amyloid and increased frequency of type 4 allele in late-onset familial Alzheimer disease. *Proc Natl Acad Sci U S A. 90*, 1977-81.

[43] Ma J, Yee A, Brewer HB Jr, Das S, Potter H. (1994) Amyloid-associated proteins alpha 1-antichymotrypsin and apolipoprotein E promote assembly of Alzheimer beta-protein into filaments. *Nature. 372*, 92-4.

[44] Goedert M, Strittmatter WJ, Roses AD. (1994) Alzheimer's disease. Risky apolipoprotein in brain. *Nature. 372*, 45-6.

[45] Seaman MN. (2005) Recycle your receptors with retromer. *Trends Cell Biol. 15*, 68-75.

[46] Jin K, Peel AL, Mao XO, Xie L, Cottrell BA, Henshall DC, Greenberg DA. (2004) Increased hippocampal neurogenesis in Alzheimer's disease. *Proc Natl Acad Sci U S A. 101*, 343-7.

[47] Feng R, Rampon C, Tang YP, Shrom D, Jin J, Kyin M, Sopher B, Miller MW, Ware CB, Martin GM, Kim SH, Langdon RB, Sisodia SS, Tsien JZ. (2001) Deficient neurogenesis in forebrain-specific presenilin-1 knockout mice is associated with reduced clearance of hippocampal memory traces. *Neuron. 32*, 911-26. Erratum in: (2002) *Neuron. 33*, 313.

[48] Wen PH, Friedrich VL Jr, Shioi J, Robakis NK, Elder GA. (2002) Presenilin-1 is expressed in neural progenitor cells in the hippocampus of adult mice. *Neurosci Lett.* 318, 53-6.

[49] Jin K, Galvan V, Xie L, Mao XO, Gorostiza OF, Bredesen DE, Greenberg DA. (2004) Enhanced neurogenesis in Alzheimer's disease transgenic (PDGF-APPSw,Ind) mice. *Proc Natl Acad Sci U S A. 101*, 13363-7.

[50] Nowakowski, RS, Lewin SB, Miller MW. (1989) Bromodeoxyuridine immunohistochemical determination of the lengths of the cell cycle and the DNA-synthetic phase for an anatomically defined population. *J. Neurocytol. 18*, 311-8.

[51] Miller MW, Nowakowski RS. (1988) Use of bromodeoxyuridine-immunohistochemistry to examine the proliferation, migration and time of origin of cells in the central nervous system. *Brain Res. 457*, 44-52.

[52] Guenette SY, Tanzi RE. (1999) Progress toward valid transgenic mouse models for Alzheimer's disease. *Neurobiol Aging. 20*, 201-11.

[53] Dodart JC, Mathis C, Bales KR, Paul SM. (2002) Does my mouse have Alzheimer's disease? *Genes Brain Behav. 1*, 142-55.

[54] Yang Y, Geldmacher DS, Herrup K. (2001) DNA replication precedes neuronal cell death in Alzheimer's disease. *J Neurosci. 21*, 2661-8.

[55] Herrup K, Neve R, Ackerman SL, Copani A. (2004) Divide and die: cell cycle events as triggers of nerve cell death. *J Neurosci. 24*, 9232-9.

[56] Nowakowski RS, Hayes NL. (2000) New neurons: extraordinary evidence or extraordinary conclusion? *Science. 288*, 771.

[57] Nowakowski RS, Hayes NL. (2001) Stem cells: the promises and pitfalls. *Neuropsychopharmacology. 25*, 799-804.

[58] Gould E, Gross CG. (2002) Neurogenesis in adult mammals: some progress and problems. *J Neurosci. 22*, 619-23.

[59] Rakic P. (2002) Adult neurogenesis in mammals: an identity crisis. *J Neurosci. 22*, 614-8.

[60] Taupin P. (2007) BrdU Immunohistochemistry for Studying Adult Neurogenesis: paradigms, pitfalls, limitations, and validation. *Brain Research Reviews. 53*, 198-214.

[61] Taupin P. (2007) Protocols for Studying Adult Neurogenesis: Insights and Recent Developments. *Regenerative Medicine. 2*, 51-62.

[62] Taupin P. (2006) Neurogenesis and Alzheimer's Disease. *Drug Target Insights. 1*, 1-4.

[63] Beghi E. (2007) Epilepsy. *Curr Opin Neurol. 20*, 169-74.

[64] Hermann B, Seidenberg M. (2007) Epilepsy and cognition. *Epilepsy Curr. 7*, 1-6.

[65] Shorvon S. (2007) The treatment of chronic epilepsy: a review of recent studies of clinical efficacy and side effects. *Curr Opin Neurol. 20*, 159-63.

[66] Arango MF, Steven DA, Herrick IA. (2004) Neurosurgery for the treatment of epilepsy. *Curr Opin Anaesthesiol. 17*, 383-7.

[67] Morrell M. (2006) Brain stimulation for epilepsy: can scheduled or responsive neurostimulation stop seizures? *Curr Opin Neurol. 19*, 164-8.

[68] Thom M. (2004) Recent advances in the neuropathology of focal lesions in epilepsy. *Expert Rev Neurother. 4*, 973-84.

[69] Collins RC, Tearse RG, Lothman EW. (1983) Functional anatomy of limbic seizures: focal discharges from medial entorhinal cortex in rat. *Brain Res. 280*, 25-40.

[70] Heinemann U, Beck H, Dreier JP, Ficker E, Stabel J, Zhang CL. (1992) The dentate gyrus as a regulated gate for the propagation of epileptiform activity. *Epilepsy Res Suppl. 7*, 273-80.

[71] Sloviter RS. (1991) Feedforward and feedback inhibition of hippocampal principal cell activity evoked by perforant path stimulation: GABA-mediated mechanisms that regulate excitability in vivo. *Hippocampus. 1*, 31-40.

[72] Houser CR. (1990) Granule cell dispersion in the dentate gyrus of humans with temporal lobe epilepsy. *Brain Res. 535*, 195-204.

[73] de Lanerolle NC, Kim JH, Robbins RJ, Spencer DD. (1989) Hippocampal interneuron loss and plasticity in human temporal lobe epilepsy. *Brain Res. 495*, 387-95.

[74] Sutula T, Cascino G, Cavazos J, Parada I, Ramirez L. (1989) Mossy fiber synaptic reorganization in the epileptic human temporal lobe. *Ann Neurol. 26*, 321-30.

[75] Represa A, Tremblay E, Ben-Ari Y. (1990) Sprouting of mossy fibers in the hippocampus of epileptic human and rat. *Adv Exp Med Biol. 268*, 419-24.

[76] Babb TL, Kupfer WR, Pretorius JK, Crandall PH, Levesque MF. (1991) Synaptic reorganization by mossy fibers in human epileptic fascia dentata. *Neurosci. 42*, 351-63.

[77] Sloviter RS. (1987) Decreased hippocampal inhibition and a selective loss of interneurons in experimental epilepsy. *Science. 235*, 73-6.

[78] Tauck DL, Nadler JV. (1985) Evidence of functional mossy fiber sprouting in hippocampal formation of kainic acid-treated rats. *J Neurosci. 5*, 1016-22.

[79] Cronin J, Dudek FE. (1988) Chronic seizures and collateral sprouting of dentate mossy fibers after kainic acid treatment in rats. *Brain Res. 474*, 181-4.

[80] Sloviter RS. (1992) Possible functional consequences of synaptic reorganization in the dentate gyrus of kainate-treated rats. *Neurosci Lett. 137*, 91-6.

[81] Longo BM, Mello LE. (1997) Blockade of pilocarpine- or kainate-induced mossy fiber sprouting by cycloheximide does not prevent subsequent epileptogenesis in rats. *Neurosci Lett. 226*, 163-6.

[82] Longo BM, Mello LE. (1998) Supragranular mossy fiber sprouting is not necessary for spontaneous seizures in the intrahippocampal kainate model of epilepsy in the rat. *Epilepsy Res. 32*, 172-82.

[83] Parent JM, Yu TW, Leibowitz RT, Geschwind DH, Sloviter RS, Lowenstein DH. (1997) Dentate granule cell neurogenesis is increased by seizures and contributes to aberrant network reorganization in the adult rat hippocampus. *J Neurosci. 17*, 3727-38.

[84] Bengzon J, Kokaia Z, Elmer E, Nanobashvili A, Kokaia M, Lindvall O. (1997) Apoptosis and proliferation of dentate gyrus neurons after single and intermittent limbic seizures. *Proc Natl Acad Sci U S A. 94*, 10432-7.

[85] Gray WP, Sundstrom LE. (1998) Kainic acid increases the proliferation of granule cell progenitors in the dentate gyrus of the adult rat. *Brain Res. 790*, 52-9.

[86] Scharfman HE, Goodman JH, Sollas AL. (2000) Granule-like neurons at the hilar/CA3 border after status epilepticus and their synchrony with area CA3 pyramidal cells: functional implications of seizure-induced neurogenesis. *J Neurosci. 20*, 6144-58.

[87] Covolan L, Ribeiro LT, Longo BM, Mello LE. (2000) Cell damage and neurogenesis in the dentate granule cell layer of adult rats after pilocarpine- or kainate-induced status epilepticus. *Hippocampus. 10*, 69-80.

[88] Cavalheiro EA, Leite JP, Bortolotto ZA, Turski WA, Ikonomidou C, Turski L. (1991) Long-term effects of pilocarpine in rats: structural damage of the brain triggers kindling and spontaneous recurrent seizures. *Epilepsia. 32*, 778-82.

[89] Mello LE, Cavalheiro EA, Tan AM, Kupfer WR, Pretorius JK, Babb TL, Finch DM. (1993) Circuit mechanisms of seizures in the pilocarpine model of chronic epilepsy: cell loss and mossy fiber sprouting. *Epilepsia. 34*, 985-95.

[90] Tauck DL, Nadler JV. (1985) Evidence of functional mossy fiber sprouting in hippocampal formation of kainic acid-treated rats. *J Neurosci. 5*, 1016-22.

[91] Cronin J, Dudek FE. (1988) Chronic seizures and collateral sprouting of dentate mossy fibers after kainic acid treatment in rats. *Brain Res. 474*, 181-4.

[92] Represa A, Ben-Ari Y. (1992) Kindling is associated with the formation of novel mossy fibre synapses in the CA3 region. *Exp Brain Res. 92*, 69-78.

[93] Sloviter RS. (1992) Possible functional consequences of synaptic reorganization in the dentate gyrus of kainate-treated rats. *Neurosci Lett. 137*, 91-6.

[94] Parent JM, Tada E, Fike JR, Lowenstein DH. (1999) Inhibition of dentate granule cell neurogenesis with brain irradiation does not prevent seizure-induced mossy fiber synaptic reorganization in the rat. *J Neurosci. 19*, 4508-19.

[95] Ferland RJ, Williams JP, Gross RA, Applegate CD. (2003) The effects of brain-irradiation-induced decreases in hippocampal mitotic activity on flurothyl-induced epileptogenesis in adult C57BL/6J mice. *Exp Neurol. 179*, 71-82.

[96] Spalding KL, Bhardwaj RD, Buchholz BA, Druid H, Frisen J. (2005) Retrospective birth dating of cells in humans. *Cell. 122*, 133-43.

[97] Bhardwaj RD, Curtis MA, Spalding KL, Buchholz BA, Fink D, Bjork-Eriksson T, Nordborg C, Gage FH, Druid H, Eriksson PS, Frisen J. (2006) Neocortical neurogenesis in humans is restricted to development. *Proc Natl Acad Sci U S A. 103*, 12564-8.

[98] Reiman EM, Webster JA, Myers AJ, Hardy J, Dunckley T, Zismann VL, Joshipura KD, Pearson JV, Hu-Lince D, Huentelman MJ, Craig DW, Coon KD, Liang WS, Herbert RH, Beach T, Rohrer KC, Zhao AS, Leung D, Bryden L, Marlowe L, Kaleem M, Mastroeni D, Grover A, Heward CB, Ravid R, Rogers J, Hutton ML, Melquist S, Petersen RC, Alexander GE, Caselli RJ, Kukull W, Papassotiropoulos A, Stephan DA. (2007) GAB2 Alleles Modify Alzheimer's Risk in APOE varepsilon4 Carriers. *Neuron. 54*, 713-20.

Conclusion and Perspectives

Over the past decades, significant progresses have been made in our understanding of the functioning, and physio- and pathology of the nervous system, particularly the hippocampus. Some of these progresses have confirmed and precise previous concepts and studies. Gene profiling of the subregions of the hippocampus has confirmed the existence of the *Cornu Ammonis* (CA) region CA2 of the hippocampus, previously defined by Lorente de No (1934) based on histological studies [1]. These studies further reveal the molecular identity of the cell types of the hippocampal regions [2].

Others have challenged basic concepts and dogma that were governing the field of neurosciences. The evidences that granule cells of the hippocampal dentate gyrus (DG) and their ending nerves, the Mossy fiber (MF) terminals, contain and release γ-aminobutyric acid (GABA) leaded to the identification of GABA, as a neurotransmitter of the MF-CA3 pyramidal cell synapse. The MF synapse is a "dual" synapse, with two "fast-acting" neurotransmitters, Glu and GABA, excitatory and inhibitory neurotransmitters, respectfively [3,4]. The depolarizing activity of GABA during development highlights the functional plasticity of the GABAergic phenotype [5].The confirmation that neurogenesis occurs in the adult brain and neural stem cells reside in the adult central nervous system (CNS) suggests that the development of the brain may never end and the CNS may be amenable to repair [6-8].

These studies have tremendous consequences for our understanding of development, functioning, physio- and pathology of the CNS, as well as for therapy. Particularly, adult neural stem cells carry a lot of potential and hope for the treatment and cure of a broad range of neurological diseases, disorders and injuries.

However, these progresses have come with more questions than answers. Recent developments in biomedical research, like the generation of a 3-dimesional atlas of the genes expressed in the brain [9] and the sequencing the macaque and chimpanzee genomes, that share 93% and 98.7% of the genome sequences with human, respectively [10,11], bring to the scientific community invaluable knowledge and tools to further unravel the mechanisms underlying brain development, functioning, physio- and pathology, and to translate basic research to therapy.

REFERENCES

[1] Lein ES, Callaway EM, Albright TD, Gage FH. (2005) Redefining the boundaries of the hippocampal CA2 subfield in the mouse using gene expression and 3-dimensional reconstruction. *J Comp Neurol. 485*, 1-10.

[2] Lorente de No R. (1934) Studies on the structure of the cerebral cortex. II. Continuation of the study of the ammonic system. *J Psychol Neurol (Lpz). 46*, 113-77.

[3] Sandler R, Smith AD. (1991) Coexistence of GABA and glutamate in mossy fiber terminals of the primate hippocampus: an ultrastructural study. *J Comp Neurol. 303*, 177-92.

[4] Taupin P, Ben-Ari Y, Roisin MP. (1994) Subcellular fractionation on Percoll gradient of mossy fiber synaptosomes: evoked release of glutamate, GABA, aspartate and glutamate decarboxylase activity in control and degranulated rat hippocampus. *Brain Res. 644*, 313-21.

[5] Ben-Ari Y. (2002) Excitatory actions of gaba during development: the nature of the nurture. *Nat Rev Neurosci. 3*, 728-39.

[6] Gage FH. (2000) Mammalian neural stem cells. *Science. 287*, 1433-8.

[7] Kaplan MS. (2001) Environment complexity stimulates visual cortex neurogenesis: death of a dogma and a research career. *Trends Neurosci. 24*, 617-20.

[8] Taupin P, Gage FH. (2002) Adult neurogenesis and neural stem cells of the central nervous system in mammals. *J Neurosci Res. 69*, 745-9.

[9] Lein ES, Hawrylycz MJ, Ao N, Ayres M, Bensinger A, et al. (2007) Genome-wide atlas of gene expression in the adult mouse brain. *Nature. 445*, 168-76.

[10] Chimpanzee Sequencing and Analysis Consortium. (2005) Initial sequence of the chimpanzee genome and comparison with the human genome. *Nature. 437*, 69-87.

[11] Rhesus Macaque Genome Sequencing and Analysis Consortium. Gibbs RA, Rogers J, Katze MG, Bumgarner R, Weinstock GM, et al. (2007) Evolutionary and biomedical insights from the rhesus macaque genome. *Science. 316*, 222-34.

INDEX

A

B

C

D

E

M

N

O

P

Q

R

S

T

U

V

W

X

Z